Developmental Nephrology

WALLACE W. McCRORY, M.D.

A COMMONWEALTH FUND BOOK

HARVARD UNIVERSITY PRESS, CAMBRIDGE, MASSACHUSETTS, 1972

To Sylvia, Heather, Sean, and Robin

This volume is published as part of a long-standing cooperative program between Harvard University Press and the Commonwealth Fund, a philanthropic foundation, to encourage the publication of significant scholarly books in medicine and health.

Preface

The anatomic and physiologic characteristics that distinguish the immature newborn kidney from the mature kidney of the adult have been extensively documented in comparative terms. This approach emphasizes the age-related differences, but it focuses on only two points of time in a growth spectrum that begins with embryogenesis and ends with senescence. Pediatrics is now concerned with the whole period of human growth and maturation and the several biologic processes involved in human development. It would be timely, therefore, to view the growth of the kidney from fetal life to adulthood from the developmental standpoint, that is, in terms of the sequential growth processes that are involved.

This developmental perspective can be achieved if we examine the changes occurring in the structure and function of the kidney during the whole period of childhood growth. We must, then, begin with embryogenesis and consider the changes occurring during the fetal period when embryogenesis and structural and functional maturation proceed pari passu. Sufficient data are now available to permit a description of renal development in fetal life and in the perinatal period from the morphologic, physiologic, and biochemical viewpoints. The perinatal period exhibits striking growth activity and unique functional changes as part of the process of adaptation to extrauterine life. The period of childhood growth is one of slow but continuous development and during this period organ function adapts to the changing work requirements. This multifaceted process can most succinctly be categorized under the rubric of *Developmental Nephrology*. This monograph is so named because it attempts to view the growth and development of the kidney as an integral part of the normal process of growth of the fetus to adulthood.

Renal embryogenesis, differentiation, and development have been reviewed to provide a basis for more fruitful exploration of the mechanisms responsible for faulty development (that is, congenital malformations). An attempt has been made to correlate data relevant to the development of the kidney from the aspect of observed changes in gross structure as well as cellular structure, function, and organization from the first appearance of the pronephros to the final appearance of the mature kidney. The data available on quantitative measurement of renal function during postnatal development have been reviewed and the gaps in our knowledge explored. A summary of the new field of research directed at definition of the mechanisms regulating renal work and renal growth has been included.

Our rapidly expanding knowledge about the molecular and cellular aspects of biology has occurred in an era of equally impressive technologic advances in methods available to investigators studying the biology of man. The tools of the morphologist have been sharpened by electron microscopy, new microhistochemical and immunochemical techniques, and reapplication of microdissection; those of the physiologist by micropuncture allowing study of the function of single nephrons, and methods for isolating functional portions of single nephrons in vitro. Biochemists can isolate subcellular components and study their structure and function with available techniques.

It is difficult, if not impossible, to keep abreast of all of the relevant and important new work and to appreciate its implications for new concepts of pathogenesis of renal disease and renal development and functional maturation. The delay time required for new ideas to gain wide familiarity in the potential community of interested health scientists is increasing at an awesome pace. It is my hope that the material collected in this monograph will provide a new perspective in some areas for those students, biologists, and physicians interested in the kidney but too involved with their special trees to notice some of the changes occurring in the forest in which they toil.

A case in point is provided by the exciting new concepts advanced by Jean Oliver in his monograph *Nephrons and Kidneys: A Quantitative*

Study of Developmental and Evolutionary Mammalian Renal Architectonics (New York: Hoeber Medical Division, Harper and Row, 1968). The reader will be rewarded in direct proportion to the time he spends with this unusual book. The architectonic concept presented by Oliver provides an integrated developmental blueprint upon which the program of normal renal development can be viewed in quantitative terms. The hypotheses advanced are sufficiently well documented to stand critical review and sufficiently revisionist to make our present concepts of the basis of renal structural maldevelopment obsolete. His work is especially valuable because it documents the normal development of the human kidney from early fetal life.

There are limits to the application that can be made of new hypotheses regarding basic biologic phenomena developed out of studies of simpler biologic models than mammals or man. The final step in the application of new biologic advances to benefit the sick child or adult always requires the direct study of mammals and ultimately of man himself. This is tedious, frustrating, and difficult—but a surprising amount of data have been accumulated by direct studies of man. I have tried to provide a comprehensive review of all of the relevant sources of data up to 1970, but I realize that we all have blind spots when we search the literature. I should appreciate having my blind spots corrected by communication from readers with better vision.

The writing of this monograph was aided by a grant-in-aid from the Commonwealth Fund, and their confidence in the potential value of this type of scholarly work was most important in initiating and sustaining my venture in preparing a book on a new area of child health. The writing was done during a sabbatical leave spent as a visiting professor at the Institute of Child Health, London, England, a privilege extended to me by a colleague and friend, Dr. Otto Wolff, Professor of Child Health, and the faculty of the Institute of Child Health, University of London. I was greatly aided in my literature research by the superb facilities of the Library of the Royal Society of Medicine, which were provided to me as a Fellow of the Royal Society of Medicine.

I wish to acknowledge with respect and appreciation the advice, stimulation, and criticism provided by a few most enjoyable sessions with Dr. Jean Oliver and I appreciate his willingness to provide original prints for inclusion in Chapter 1. I was fortunate in having the encouragement and unique secretarial services of my wife, Sylvia Hogben McCrory, during the long period this book was "aborning" as well as her uncomplaining indulgence as quiet hours went by. I also wish to thank Miss Karlusa Kovarik for her very able editorial assistance in preparing the final manuscript.

W. W. McC.

Contents

TABLES

FIGURES

PLATES (following page 50)

Developmental Nephrology

Chapter 1. Embryologic Development of the Kidney

The embryologic development of the human kidney can be viewed as a goal-oriented program aimed at achievement of the unique anatomic configuration responsible for the aggregate functional efficiency of its 1,000,000 nephrons. The relations between organ form and function are nowhere more superbly illustrated than by examination of the differentiation and development of the kidney. The kidney of man is more complex than that of the rat, dog, or ape. The bases underlying the unique form and function of the adult human kidney become evident when we consider its embryology. As a first step let us examine briefly both ontologic and phylogenetic aspects of mammalian renal development as a prologue to describing renal organogenesis in man.

The fascinating evolutionary speculations of Oliver[1] provide some insight into the differences in definitive architectonic patterns found in various mammalian kidney types and suggest that they can be comprehended as the result of two different ontogenetic and phylogenetic responses to the continuous biologic requirement for some kind of parity between kidney size and body size.

The major architectonic differences between mammalian kidneys are most obvious in the two extremes of mammalian size: the small shrew with a unipapillary kidney and the giant whale with a multirenculated kidney. The size of the mammal, however, does not determine the type of kidney, since the horse and camel also have a unipapillary kidney. Oliver proposes that two independent adaptive organ growth processes, functional adaptation and environmental selection of mutations, can be viewed as operating differently in various species to influence one or the other of the two major architectonic determinants of ultimate kidney configuration, the growth of the nephrons and the collecting-duct system. In his view, the multirenculated human kidney arose as a result of the selection of a *mutational change* of the duct system involving its early division which led to the multilobed kidney with its multicalycine-ductal complex. The early divisions of the ductal complex set the program for the development of a multilobed kidney. The crest kidney found in the horse and camel is an example of how the unipapillary kidney has undergone *adaptive growth modification by nephron enlargement* during evolutionary history.

Recognition of these two major architectonic differences in the pattern of mammalian kidneys is of prime importance if one is to appreciate that the order and position in which the nephrons are assembled to form the aggregate renal mass determine, in part, the functional efficiency of the composite kidney. Renal functional efficiency is determined not by number of nephrons alone, but also by how they are organized to form the kidneys.

The dimensions and relations of its individual nephrons also determine the functional efficiency of the kidney, since rates of filtration and fluid flow and membrane transport (active and passive) are dependent on physical factors such as surface area and membrane thickness. The human kidney could not function efficiently if it consisted of just two giant nephrons, because of the physical limits to the size a functionally effective nephron can assume. The capacity for adaptive growth[2] of nephrons by cell hyperplasia and compensatory hypertrophy stimulated by environmental changes and resulting in increased renal mass provides the physiologic mechanism whereby the kidney can respond when stressed by a change in functional load. This mechanism is called into play whenever structural-functional equilibrium is disturbed either by the reduction in renal mass (loss of existing renal tissue) or by an increase in work load (for example, an increase in body size with growth).

This process, however, must operate within fixed limits with respect to the functional consequences of renal compensatory growth. The success or failure of this compensatory readjustment is dependent on the number of nephron units that can participate in the structural and functional transformations that occur. When there has been too great a loss of neph-

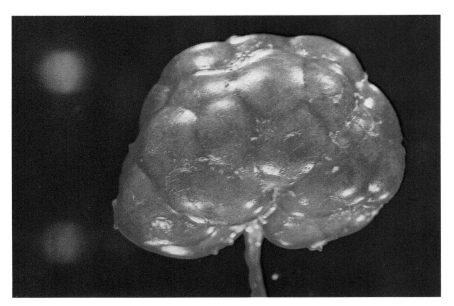

FIGURE 1.1A   Normal kidney of a newborn full-term infant, age 5 days. The individual renculi can be distinguished as lobulations visible on the lateral surface.

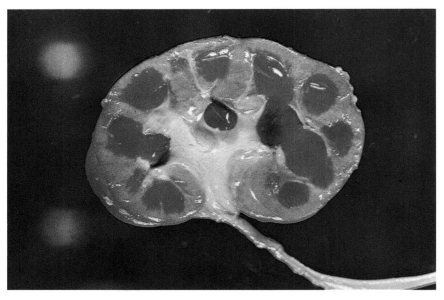

FIGURE 1.1B   Cut section, normal kidney of a newborn full-term infant, age 5 days. Some papillae can be seen projecting into minor calyces. The fusion of three papillae into a single compound structure is visible emptying into the inferior calyceal system. The pelvocalyceal system is still attached with a short section of ureter.

ron units in man (as in chronic renal disease), the result even with maximal hypertrophy is functionally inefficient and was so characterized by Oliver in his Ramon Guiteras Memorial Lecture to urologists in 1950, "When is the kidney not a kidney?"[3] Experimental studies have demonstrated the pathophysiologic validity of this concept.

Experimental reduction of renal mass in normal rats was employed by Platt, Roscoe, and Smith[4] to reproduce many of the typical phenomena of human chronic renal failure. This animal model has since become the classic one for the experimental study of these relationships. Platt and his co-workers demonstrated that when five-sixths of the kidney tissue of the adult rat was removed, the compensatory hypertrophy of the residuum could not maintain adequate renal function to support normal life because of the low operational efficiency of the remaining hypertrophied nephrons. This also applies to the young growing subject. Similar experiments in postweanling rats by Morrison[5] showed that growth failure and death from chronic renal failure occurred before maturation. These observations indicate that if we are to understand the importance of the interrelationships between structure and function we must, as Platt said, "think in terms of nephrons rather than kidneys."[6]

Correlative studies of this kind have been most productive in studies of the pathophysiology of renal failure. The functional consequences of reduction in nephron numbers through disease processes has been extensively studied and reviewed by Bricker and his associates.[7] These interrelationships have not, however, been sufficiently well defined during normal renal development to provide the necessary basis for similar studies of gross malformations of kidney structure. The morphologic appearance of the kidney is still the main basis for such classification.[8] The importance of combining quantitative functional and anatomic measurements in new attempts at analysis of structural renal malformations was emphasized in a recent review by Bernstein.[9] The investigator seeking to define such aspects can now more profitably pursue this approach because of the quantitative data made available in Oliver's monumental contribution, cited previously,[1] on the development of the normal human kidney.

This brief introduction is presented to emphasize the need for studies of renal development relating structural changes and number and function of the nephrons rather than considering structure or function alone. A brief review of the gross anatomy of the mature kidney will be presented before we undertake a detailed description of its embryologic development.

ANATOMY OF THE MATURE KIDNEY

Gross Structure

The quantitative aspects of gross kidney structure have long been known. The kidney of man is a multilobed (multirenculated) structure consisting of a cluster of renculi (average 8, range 4 to 11) that terminate in conical papillae emptying into a common calyceal-pelvic complex. The fact that the adult kidney is multilobed is nowhere better appreciated than when one observes the prominence of the lobulations on the surface of the kidney of the normal full-term newborn, as in Fig. 1.1. The lobulation disappears in infancy as cortical growth of nephrons obliterates the "grooves."

The average number of papillae found in the human kidney is 8 (range 4 to 11).[10] The occurrence of two or three papillae fused into a compound structure is not uncommon, as seen in Fig. 1.1, and in counts of papillae this must be given consideration. Each renculus is organized as a self-contained functional unit that consists of a mantle of cortical tissue whose nephrons drain into a confluence of collecting ducts that form the base of the medullary pyramids which end in a papilla. The mantle of cortical tissue surrounds the medullary base in the manner of a cap-like shell, and some cortical tissue extends laterally down the side of the pyramids projecting into the medullary space between the pyramids (the renal columns of Bertin). The confluence of collecting ducts terminates in the ducts of Bellini in the renal papillae. These can be enumerated as individual pores in the area cribrosa (average number 44 ± 15). In attempts to define gross renal structure, counting the ducts of Bellini can be of value in recognizing compound papillae.

Malformations associated with quantitative abnormalities in the number of lobes (renculi) or pyramids have been described in man. In one form known as the Ask-Upmark kidney there appears to be unilateral segmental hypoplasia associated with hypertension in childhood.[11] Royer and his associates[12] have described another form with bilateral renal hypoplasia in which many specimens contain a reduced number of pyramids; even unirencular and birencular kidneys have been observed. There is a greatly reduced number of nephrons, and those present are remarkably hypertrophied (oligomeganephronie). These examples of developmental malformations associated with a reduced number of renculi or pyramids could be the result of anomalous early branching of the ureteric bud.

Variations of Cortical and Medullary Nephron Size in the Mature Kidney

While the average glomerular diameter is fairly uniform (100 microns), in different areas of the mature kidney there are differences in physical dimensions of the various tubular parts of the nephrons that are related to their location in the different levels of the cortex. If one arbitrarily divides the cortex into three zones—inner, middle, and outer—with respect to their proximity to the medulla, the proximal tubules of nephrons tend to be longest in the outer zone and shortest in the inner zone, with a mean overall length of about 20 mm. They vary in length from 12 to 24 mm and from 50 to 65 microns in external diameter. The thin limbs vary from 0 to 14 mm in length and 14 to 22 microns in diameter. The thick limbs of Henle's loop vary from 6 to 18 mm in length. The distal convoluted segments vary in length from 2 to 9 mm and 20 to 50 microns in diameter. The total length of nephrons is difficult to define in absolute terms because of the great variation in the length of arcades comprised of fused nephronic segments (or connecting tubules). The total length of nephrons excluding collecting ducts has been found to vary from 20 to 44 mm. The average length of the collecting ducts is 22 mm, and their external diameters may be as large as 200 microns at their termination at the ducts of Bellini.[13]

The proximal tubules account for the bulk of renal parenchyma. The cortical nephrons lying in the outer two-thirds of the cortex (seven-eighths of all nephrons) have relatively short loops of Henle. Some lie entirely within the cortex and have no thin segments, while others penetrate the medulla to varying depths. They usually have short thin segments or none at all. The nephrons lying in the inner third of the cortex (about one-eighth of all nephrons) constitute the juxtamedullary nephrons. They have long well-developed loops and the thin segments of some loops extend into the tips of the papillae. The proportion of nephrons in the kidney possessing long well-developed loops of Henle is of great functional significance since it is known that the mammalian capacity to form urine of high solute content requires the presence of nephrons with long loops of Henle. Those mammals with the greatest capacity to concentrate urinary solute (desert rodents) have only nephrons with very long loops of Henle.[13]

The distal convoluted tubules are joined to their collecting ducts via *connecting tubules* that have dark granular cells which are presumably of nephronic* origin, intermixed with clear cells that resemble those of the collecting ducts (cuboidal, sparsely granular, and uniform in size) which arise from ureteral bud tissue. Collecting ducts in the outer cortex receive two or more connecting tubules. There is a confluence of collecting-duct branches as they course through the cortex toward the medulla, where they finally form the papillary ducts which drain into the minor calyces.

It was once thought that the collecting tubules played no significant role in the formation of the final composition of urine. This view held that after tubular fluid left the distal convoluted tubule there was little alteration in its composition during its subsequent transit through the collecting system. There is now clear evidence that the collecting ducts share some of the functional attributes of the distal convoluted tubules,[16] but this portion of the renal tubular system still escapes precise functional definition.

The ultrastructure of the various portions of the adult nephron will not be described here since this information is readily available in the current literature. Certain aspects of morphologic detail have been selected for comment because of their special relevance to a systematic understanding of the normal growth processes directing renal development.

* Terminology used to describe the various parts of the nephron varies among morphologists and physiologists partly because they approach the task of nomenclature from positions of different orientation—the former configurational, the latter stressing functional specificity. Oliver's approach, because of his choice of the technique of microdissection, provides a unique way to observe the exact relations of the constituent nephrons and collecting ducts during all stages of renal development in man. The generally accepted nomenclature found in contemporary textbooks stemming from the work of Peter[14] and Felix[15] designates the termination of the distal nephron to be at its transition to the connecting tubule which is part of the collecting-tubule system; hence it would originate from ureteral bud tissue and not from the nephronic vesicle. Italics are used throughout the text to denote Oliver's terminology. Oliver presents convincing evidence that the connecting tubule is of nephronic origin, arising from tissue differentiating from the induced nephronic vesicle rather than the ductal system. The recognition of the number of legitimate progeny of the ureteral bud and nephronic vesicle is one of Oliver's major contributions, and familiarity with his distinctions between collecting ducts and nephrons is fundamental to understanding his description of renal development in quantitative terms.

The Renal Vascular System

The renal arteries usually arise from the aorta opposite the upper border of the second lumbar vertebra, the right passing posterior to the inferior vena cava. Approaching the hilus, they divide into anterior and posterior branches to specific parts of the renal parenchyma. As the various segmental arteries penetrate the renal parenchyma, they branch into interlobular arteries which penetrate the renal columns and pass between adjacent pyramids. At the corticomedullary junction each interlobular artery divides dichotomously into branches known as arcuate arteries, which pass along the corticomedullary boundary parallel to the capsule sending off intralobular branches to supply the nephrons.

The vascular supply of the cortical nephrons is quite different from that of the juxtamedullary nephrons (see Fig. 1.2). The efferent arteriole of the cortical nephrons is slightly smaller than the afferent and breaks up immediately to form a freely anastomosing network of capillaries that envelops the proximal and distal convolutions and the portions of the ascending and descending limbs of Henle's loop and collecting ducts in the cortical zone. These capillary networks recombine into venules which join to form interlobular veins.

In the juxtamedullary nephrons the efferent arteriole is of equal or greater diameter than the afferent. It gives off branches that form an anastomosing network of capillaries supplying the cortical proximal and distal convolutions in a pattern similar to that found in the cortex. In addition to the supply to this network, however, it sends repeated arteriolar branches that penetrate into the medulla, following the descending limbs of Henle's loop to the tip of the medulla, as in Fig. 1.2. These vessels turn with the bend of Henle's loop and return to the corticomedullary junction, reassembling into venules which enter the interlobular veins close to their junction with an arcuate vein.

These straight and vertically aligned vessels form the *vasa recta*, and the hairpin arrangement allows them to function as countercurrent exchangers while providing the blood supply of the medulla. The blood flowing through the vasa recta bypasses the proximal tubules. The functional significance of the hairpin configuration of the loops of Henle and anatomic differences in blood supply between cortical and medullary regions of the kidney are described in detail in other sources.[17] The renal cortex has a much higher rate of blood flow per gram of the tissue than the renal medulla. Since the cortex accounts for about three-fourths of total kidney tissue perfused, most of the renal blood flow perfuses the

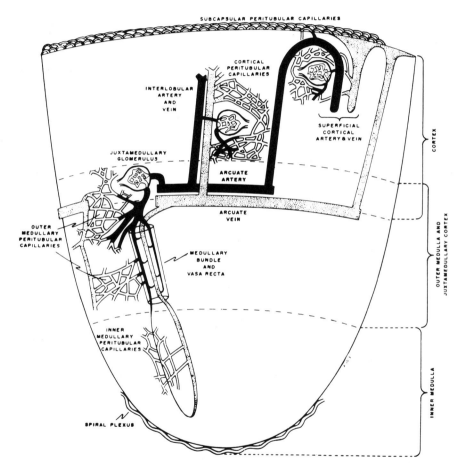

FIGURE 1.2 Vascular supply of the cortical and juxtamedullary nephrons. The efferent arteriole in the cortical nephrons breaks down into a network of peritubular capillaries that surround the proximal convoluted tubules. The efferent arteriole of the juxtamedullary glomeruli forms a similar plexus but also sends other direct arteriolar branches down into the medulla before branching, forming vasa recta and supplying the tissues of the inner medulla. (From Pomeranz, Birtch, and Barger.[20])

renal cortex. The importance of slow medullary blood flow for maintenance of renal concentrating ability has been emphasized by Thurau.[18]

The intrarenal distribution of blood flow may vary under different physiologic conditions. Horster and Thurau[19] performed micropuncture studies which demonstrated that a disparity can be observed between values for filtration rates in single superficial cortical and deep (juxtamedullary) glomeruli in the rat kidney in certain situations. They found that the value for glomerular filtration rate in superficial single nephrons was lower than that found in juxtamedullary single nephrons in rats during antidiuresis and when on salt-poor diets.

The distribution of intrarenal blood flow is under neural control in the dog. Pomeranz, Birtch, and Barger[20] have shown that mild renal nerve stimulation in dogs, while not necessarily altering total renal blood flow, decreases perfusion of the outer cortical peritubular capillaries and increases flow to the outer medulla and juxtamedullary nephrons (Fig. 1.2). These changes could also be produced by intra-arterial injection of norephinephrine and reversed by adrenergic vasodilatation. Redistribution of blood flow was shown to correlate well with sodium excretion. Conditions which redistribute flow from cortex to outer medulla cause increased sodium resorption, and conversely conditions which increase cortical flow and decrease outer medullary flow promote sodium excretion. Several possible hypotheses were proposed by the authors to explain how neurogenic redistribution of intrarenal blood flow may promote sodium resorption—including the possibility that redistribution of filtrate from outer cortical nephrons with short loops of Henle to inner nephrons with long loops promotes sodium resorption. The relevance of these observations to the human kidney has not yet been documented.

ORIGIN OF THE METANEPHROS

The kidney in man arises through a process that is described in standard textbooks of embryology as one that involves the differentiation of three different paired organs composed of histologically different nephron structures, of which only the last persists and develops during fetal growth to function as the definitive excretory organ in mammals throughout life.[21,22]

The development of the mammalian kidney thus differs from most viscera, such as the liver. In the latter case, the organ evolves by a direct continuous process beginning with and incorporating an initial anlage.

In the case of the kidney, two primitive excretory organs (designated as the pronephros and mesonephros) first appear and then disappear; they might seem to be abortive trials of organogenesis, but in reality they play a vital role in the process responsible for differentiation of the third and final excretory organ that remains, the metanephros. The ontogenetic process of the kidney has significant phylogenetic interest, since a structure similar to the pronephros persists as the functional kidney in amphioxus, in the cyclostomae, and in larval forms of certain primitive fishes—as does the mesonephros in most anamniotes (fishes and amphibians). Only the amniotes (reptiles, birds, and mammals) possess a metanephros.[23]

The pronephros in man is a rudimentary nonfunctional kidney that appears and undergoes complete involution within two weeks. Its first anlage appears about the middle of the third week and its regression is completed by the fifth week; its only functional remnant is the pronephric duct. Torrey has shown in detailed studies on very early human embryos[24] that the first group of individual paired tubules of the pronephros arises as single nephrotomes in solid masses of cells of mesoblastic origin at the level of the seventh somite. Each nephrotome hollows out, but the resulting vesicle fails to differentiate into a true nephron; its external pole gives rise to a tubular bud which grows out caudally and finally fuses with the tubular bud of the next nephrotome. The tube thus formed, which is called the pronephric duct, extends past the seventh somite and finally reaches the cloaca at the end of the fourth week (Figs. 1.3A and B).

Beyond somite 7 individualized nephrotomes are no longer found, but instead a nephrogenic blastema. This bears a longitudinal cleft dividing it into a narrow lateral nephric duct and a larger medial portion, the nephrogenic cord. Seven nephrons arise from this cord, which later open into the preexisting nephric duct. These very rudimentary nephrons as described by Torrey are comprised of a capsule with a flat visceral epithelium enclosing the glomerulus vascularized by a branch of the dorsal aorta. The periglomerular space opens at one end into the coelom through a narrow peritoneal funnel (the nephrostome) and the tubule opens at the other end into the nephric duct (Fig. 1.3B). The nephrons of the mesonephros also arise from the nephrogenic cord. They cease forming nephrostomes but continue to establish union with the nephric duct. Viewed topographically, the pronephros is a cervical organ while the mesonephros is a thoracic kidney.

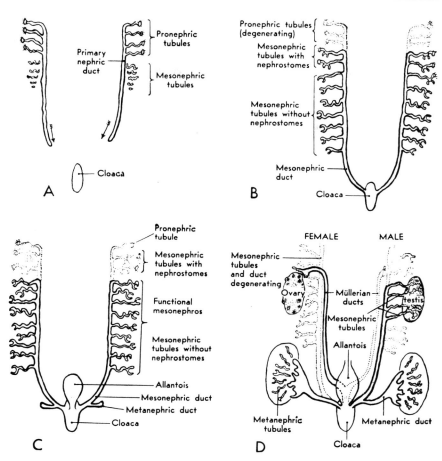

FIGURE 1.3 Schematic diagrams to show the relations of pronephros, meso-nephros, and metanephros at various stages of development. For the sake of simplicity, the tubules have been drawn as if they had been pulled out to the side of the ducts. The plan, as shown in *C,* represents approximately the conditions attained by the human embryo toward the end of the fourth week. In *D* are depicted the conditions after sexual differentiation has taken place; female left side, male right side of the diagram. The Müllerian ducts (shown in *D*) arise in human embryos during the eighth week, in close association with the mesonephric ducts. The Müllerian ducts are the primordial tubes from which the oviducts, uterus, and vagina of the female are formed. Note that although both mesonephric and Müllerian ducts appear in all young embryos, the Müllerian ducts become vestigial in the male and the mesonephric ducts become vestigial in the female. (From B. M. Patten.[22])

The mesonephros develops in intimate relation to the nephric or Wolf-fian duct[23] in the nephrogenic cord that now extends from somites 9–10 to somites 28–29. It overlaps with the caudal part of the pronephros. The first vesicles of the mesonephros differentiate at the cranial extremity (on the twenty-fourth to twenty-fifth day). By the fifth week the cranial nephrons are already degenerating, while the caudal nephrons are just differentiating, as shown in Fig. 1.4. The Wolffian body (or meso-nephros) which is comprised of 30 to 34 nephrons at any one time thus appears to be migrating from the sixth to ninth week in a caudal direc-tion. The mesonephros disappears completely during the third month though some of its elements persist (see Fig. 1.3D). As mesonephric tubules develop, they acquire an arterial blood supply from small arteries arising from the ventrolateral aspect of the aorta. A primitive glomerulus is formed with an efferent vessel that makes a capillary plexus around the tubule. When completed the Malpighian corpuscle resembles that of the metanephros, though larger. The tubule has convolutions and an apical brush border, but there is no loop of Henle or differentiated distal segment.[23]

Formation of the metanephros can be observed at about the fifth week of fetal life. Its development is dependent on the chemical interaction of a newly formed duct-tissue offshoot called the ureteric bud (arising from the mesonephric duct) with the undifferentiated mesenchymal cell masses comprising the contiguous nephrogenic ridges (Fig. 1.5). The diverticulum forming the ureteric bud appears at about the fifth week near the caudal end of the mesonephric duct, close to its entrance into the cloaca (see Fig. 1.3C). As this bud grows upward into the nephro-genic ridges, it represents the primitive ureter of the metanephric kidney. It comes in contact with the nephrogenic ridge by cranial growth; the tip enlarges and begins to divide to start the formation of the calyces and early divisions of the collecting ducts, as shown in Fig. 1.3D. The formation of the nephrons that will ultimately constitute the metanephric kidney has now begun.

The induction of nephronic element formation starts shortly after the ureteric bud begins dividing to create major branches which ultimately form the major and minor calyces. Subsequent division of the ureteric bud eventually forms the whole tree-like branching system of collecting ducts of the kidney, with induction of nephrons proceeding simul-taneously. The stimulation of nephrogenic mesenchyme to differentiate and form nephron structures typical of either the mesonephros or the metanephros is dependent on the nature of the inducer tissue, as will

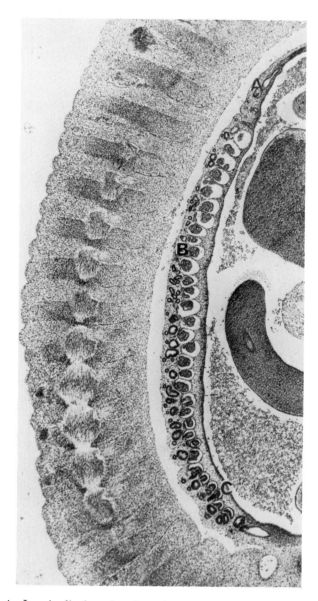

FIGURE 1.4   Longitudinal section through the mesonephros. *A*—rostral extremity, which has partly degenerated; *B*—middle portion, with differentiated nephrons; *C*—caudal extremity, still undergoing differentiation. Human embryo, 7 mm, thirty-seventh to thirty-eighth day. Magnification: x55. Institute of Anatomy, Basel. (From A. M. Du Bois.[23])

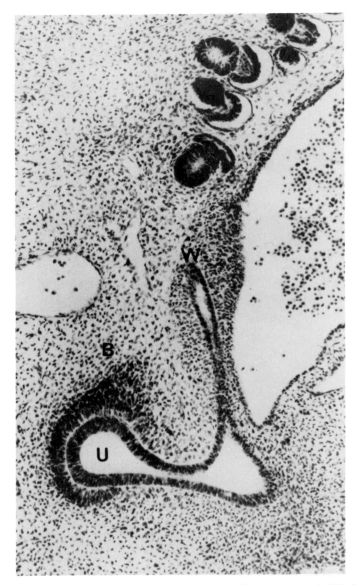

FIGURE 1.5 Caudal extremity of the mesonephros. *U*—ureteric bud; *W*—Wolffian duct; *B*—nephrogenic blastema. Human embryo, 7 mm, thirty-seventh to thirty-eighth day. Magnification: x105. Institute of Anatomy, Basel. (From A. M. Du Bois.[23])

be discussed later. The interaction of the ureteric bud and the nephrogenic blastema is necessary for differentiation of the metanephric kidney.

The development of the metanephric kidney is thus the culmination of a process of differentiation that begins with the formation of rudimentary tubular structures of no functional consequence (the pronephros) but of vital ontogenic significance. It seems somewhat artificial to attempt to separate the pronephric, mesonephric, and metanephric stages of this process. They could as easily be viewed as successive stages of a continuous morphogenetic process. Studies of precursor rudimentary organs such as the mammalian pronephros and mesonephros to define relationships between function and structure from a comparative standpoint are exceedingly complex. The value of organ systems with such a "tripartite relationship" for studies to define the control mechanisms for differentiation and organ growth and development, however, appears to be unique.*

* The term "metanephros" is usually used to distinguish this organ morphologically and functionally from the more primitive excretory organ of lower vertebrates. Investigators whose major focus is the comparative embryogenesis of the excretory system in mammals and lower vertebrates choose to consider this phenomenon as one involving the development and regression of a series of three definitive excretory organs.[25] Their approach views the development of the metanephric kidney as a product of the successive "rise and fall" of two fully functional precursor nephric organs before the third and final organ appears and persists.

There is ontogenetic justification for this view of renal development, since certain elements of the earliest "nephric tissue" originating (that is, differentiating) in mammals must be present, though in modified form, to initiate differentiation of the metanephric kidney, and some of the earlier tissues persist as other structures (such as the vas deferens). The practice of defining these as three distinct excretory organs has some usefulness, but controversy continues over the choice of suitable terms. Fraser[26] questions the validity of using the term "pronephros" or "mesonephros" for primitive mammalian embryonal structures that do not function in a manner comparable to that found when these primitive organs serve as true functional renal excretory organs. Torrey[24] suggests that the terms be used as intergrading forms of the holonephros.

As a consequence, there is an ongoing epistemologic dialogue debating the value of the concept of a "holonephros" in contrast to the "tripartite" concept of the developing kidney. The settlement of conflicting views by semantics rather than reason is not unknown in science but it has distinct perils of its own. Witness the result of a semantically related problem concerning another famous triad, belief in the Trinity. A conflict arose among theologians because of differing points of view as to the existence of a single God as opposed to three forms that share divinity. The holistic concept of one God was expanded by theologians of the western church to embrace the concept of a Trinity to resolve subtle differentiations separating God the Father, Son, and Holy Ghost. The Trinity was considered a superior device since it resolved the conflict about the essence of these three divine personages by

The blood supply in the early fetal life (8 to 19.5 mm embryo) of the mesonephros and the adjacent indeterminate cell masses is provided by a series of nonsegmental splanchnic arteries which extend laterally from the aorta. Felix[15] divides these vessels into three groups: a cranial group which passes dorsal to the adrenal gland, a middle group which passes into the adrenal gland, and a caudal group which passes ventral to the adrenal. This last group of vessels forms a plexus, the rete urogenitale, that lies between the ventral surface of the developing metanephros and the dorsal aspect of the gonad. In its early stages the metanephros may derive its blood supply from the mesonephric arteries or the rete urogenitale, but gradually three major arterial channels are formed that persist as the adrenal, renal, and gonadal arteries. The main channel of the renal artery is clearly distinguishable in the 46 mm human fetus. The renal veins are derived in large part from the supracardinal anastomosis.

The embryologic development of the metanephric kidney can thus be visualized as the end result of a complex set of interactions that involve successive steps of biochemically directed differentiation of many separate embryonic tissues. The potential for faulty interaction is great, and the result of failure of regression of formed structures or failure of induction of new structures and its relation to the production of malformations is self-evident. Failure of degeneration of pronephric tubules has been held to result in certain congenital cysts of the mediastinum. Faulty degeneration of the mesonephros accompanied by lack of resorption of the mesonephric duct has been reported in the occurrence of aberrant "ureters" emptying into a persistent Wolffian duct. Failure of the ureteric bud to divide or differentiate properly could result in renal agenesis, hypoplasia, or multicystic dysplasia with ureteric atresia.[9]

The need for appreciation of normal organogenesis to facilitate understanding of malformations of the kidney and the frequently associated malformations of the reproductive system has been so elegantly and succinctly stated by Kissane that it is quotable at this point:

combining them into one conceptual godhead, albeit with three forms. I am indebted to Professor Lancelot Hogben for acquainting me with an authentic statement of the result of this theologic synthesis in the form of the Athanasian Creed. Any scientist who has read the Athanasian Creed[27] and struggled at all to comprehend the riddles of its sophistry would not encourage any further effort to develop a comparable solution to accommodate the different points of view on renal differentiation.

If the mesomeric mesenchyme on one side is so defective (either in the strictly morphological sense or in more subtle "functional" aspects) that the pronephric duct fails to form, there will then be no structure (mesonephric duct) from which the ureteric bud can develop. In such a case, one would find not only unilateral renal agenesis but also, in the male, absence of the epididymis and ductus deferens, and in the female, absence of the inconstant epoophoron, paroophoron, and Gärtner's duct. (Demonstration of this last structure, present in perhaps 25 percent of females, requires more thorough dissection of the reproductive organs than is usually performed.) In the presence of such a basic defect in mesomeric mesenchyme, one not only would expect the homolateral gonad often to be absent but also would not be surprised to find the homolateral lung and adrenal gland to be absent as well since portions of these organs derive from the mesomere. If the lungs, adrenal glands, gonads, and sex ducts (in either sex) are all present and normally formed, one would be obliged to attribute renal agenesis to a fault in ontogeny that occurred much later, either from failure of the ureteric bud to arise from the mesonephric duct (often in association with malformations of the urogenital sinus) or from refractoriness of metanephrogenic mesenchyme to normal induction. Optimal interpretation of renal malformations, therefore, requires information regarding not only the kidneys, pelves, and ureters but also the presence, position, and state of differentiation of the gonads, sex ducts, and inconstant genital vestiges, as well as of the lungs, adrenal glands, and hindgut. Regrettably, these details are not always included in descriptions of renal malformations.[28]

ORIGIN OF THE URINARY TRACT

The differentiation of the urinary tract is synchronous with the earliest period of metanephric development. The urinary tract (extending from the renal pelvis to the external urethra) arises from a series of interactions involving a number of separate embryonic tissues. The ureters are derived from the primitive ureteric bud. The mesonephric duct, allantois, and tail gut communicate with the cloaca initially; but as development proceeds, the urinary system separates from the primitive gut when the urorectal fold forms a septum (Figs. 1.6A and B) about the sixth week

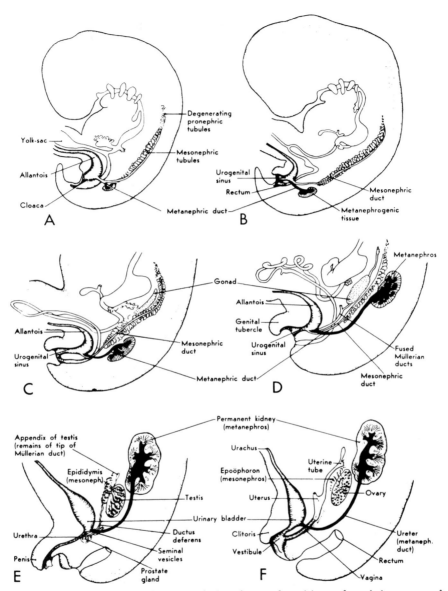

FIGURE 1.6 Diagrams showing relative sizes and positions of nephric organs of the human embryo at various stages of development. *A*—early in fifth week. (Adapted from several sources covering 5 to 6 mm embryos.) *B*—early in sixth week. (Modified from Shikinami's 8 mm embryo.) *C*—Seventh week. (Modified from Shikinami's 14.6 mm embryo.) *D*—Eighth week. (Adapted from Shikinami's 23 mm embryo and the Kelly and Burnam 25 mm stage.) *E*—male at about 3 months, schematized. *F*—female at about 3 months, schematized. (From B. M. Patten.[22])

to isolate the urogenital sinus from the rectum. The urogenital sinus is the common primordium for the bladder and the urethra.

A separate opening of the ureter directly into the urogenital sinus and lateral to that of the mesonephric duct forms through the disappearance of the terminal segment of the mesonephric duct (that short length between the termination in the cloaca and the entry of the ureter); it is incorporated into the developing bladder, which first appears as a dilatation of the urogenital sinus (Figs. 1.6C and D).

The fate of the mesonephric ducts and the mesonephric tubules differs in the two sexes from here on (Figs. 1.6E and F). In the male, the most cranial portion of the mesonephric ducts (now the Wolffian ducts) forms the highly convoluted duct of the epididymis, while the caudal portion forms the vas deferens and ejaculatory ducts and seminal vesicle. Some of the most cranial mesonephric tubules persist and become the efferent ductules of the epididymis of the adjacent developing testis. The mesonephric duct degenerates in the female, but some of the mesonephric tubules in the upper part of the mesonephros occasionally establish connections with the rete ovarii to form small usually vestigial structures known as epoophoron and paraoophoron and Gärtner's duct.

The separation of the ureters from the Wolffian ducts (as outlined above) results in formation of the trigonal area of the bladder, demarcated by the ureteric orifices and the veramontanum where the ejaculatory ducts will enter. This occurs between the eighth week (23 mm embryo) and the ninth week (35 mm embryo). The upper portion of the bladder is formed from the allantois (urachus), which ultimately contracts above the bladder to form a fibrous cord. It is rarely a significant structure at birth, but when obstructive malformations of the lower urinary tract are present it can remain patent and allow the discharge of urine to occur at the umbilicus (patent urachus).

The fetal ureter is a relatively straight tube until about the fourth month of fetal life. After this it shows two relative dilatations, one in the lumbar region between the pelviureteric junction and the ureteral crossing of the umbilical arteries and a pelvic one before its vesical insertion. This variation in caliber is not important as a factor causing congenital hydroureter. It is a reflection of the condition in utero and is not evident after birth.[29] This developmental structural adaptation may explain why the ureter of the young infant is more readily dilated by obstruction than the relatively rigid ureter of the adult and why dilatation in the infant may be of two distinct types, one involving the pelvic segment first and one in which changes in the lumbar region predominate.

The ureter of the developing metanephric kidney (secretory activity possible after the sixth week) does not open functionally into the urogenital sinus until after the 35 mm stage, or ninth week. In embryos younger than the 35 mm stage a definite membrane can be seen to stretch across the anatomic junction of the ureter and the urogenital sinus, as first shown by Chwalle[30] and verified by Gyllensten.[31] Williams[29] found that this membrane was always present in embryos of 15 to 35 mm stage and disappeared in those over 35 mm. He demonstrated such a membrane with a visible small cavity on the ureteric side in an embryo of 22 mm (eight weeks). Urine formed prior to this time would enter the cloacal cavity via the mesonephric duct. This cavity is closed distally by the cloacal membrane but is continuous with the allantoic duct. Fetal urine produced by both the mesonephros and the metanephros enters the allantoic space (Fig. 1.6A) via the urachus until its closure in the sheep and pig, but not in man where the allantois is only rudimentary. Urine formed in man would be discharged into the amniotic cavity after the cloacal membrane opens during the eighth to ninth week.

The opening of this membrane coincides in time with the onset of renal function. This was established by Gersh,[32] who correlated evidence of morphologic differentiation with evidence of tubular function and observed that tubular function begins in the human at about 32 mm or the ninth week. Chwalle[30] was of the opinion that persistence of this membrane until a later period in fetal life could result in ureterovesicular (U-V) obstruction with dilatation of the ureter above and formation of diverticulum at the site of the U-V orifice or formation of a ureterocele. Giroud[33] has shown that if the outflow of urine by the fetal kidney of the rat is temporarily impeded by experimentally induced delayed opening of epithelial septa at the ureteral openings into the primitive bladder, there can be profound dysgenetic consequences in the newborn rat—including hydronephrosis and hydroureters without evident anatomic urinary-tract obstruction at birth.

This interesting observation raises the possibility that similar transitory obstructions during embryologic development of the urinary system in man could be a factor accounting for functional urinary-tract obstructive disorders in infants associated with enlargement of the bladder and ureters (megacystic and megaureters) without demonstrable anatomic obstruction at the U-V junction or bladder outlet. The frequently noted association in the human of renal parenchymal maldevelopment with congenital anatomic obstruction of the urinary outflow tract indicates that urinary-tract obstruction occurring during renal differentiation and development can have profound effects in man. Bernstein[9] has summarized clinicopathologic and experimental data that provide evidence that fetal urinary-tract obstruction can result in embryonic malformations involving glomeruli, nephrons, and the collecting system as well as the ureteropelvocalyceal system. The hydrostatic pressure generated by the urine formed by secretory activity of the developing metanephros prior to the opening of the ureter into the developing bladder could also play a role in "modeling" the renal pelvis and calcyces of the mature kidney, although there is no direct evidence to support this hypothesis.

ORIGIN OF THE NEPHRONIC ELEMENTS OF THE METANEPHROS

The nephronic elements, or secretory parts, of the metanephric kidney arise independently of the collecting ducts but require physical association with duct tissue for successful differentiation. The mechanism of differentiation of the pronephros is unknown, but it gives rise to the Wolffian duct which, like its progeny the ureteric bud, has the capacity to induce nephron formation in mesenchyme with a nephrogenic potential. The interdependence of these different events underlying normal organogenesis of the kidney is impressive. The inhibition of the tissue differentiation involved in the early successive steps leading to the final interaction of the ureteric bud tissue with nephrogenic mesenchyme prevents the later development of the metanephros.

The developing kidney has been extensively used as a model for some of the most productive and fundamental studies of the processes regulating organogenesis. The validity of the concept of embryonic induction first proposed by Spemann[34] has been established in part by direct observations of the developing kidney. The techniques of tissue culture have been elegantly employed by Grobstein[35] and Wolff, Wolff, and Bishop-Calame,[36] and their data help explain many of the problems in its organogenesis. The description of this subject by Wolff and his co-workers should be read by those desiring a more detailed review of this subject.

The kidney arises from epithelial and mesenchymal tissues that can be separated and reassociated. This technique has been used to demonstrate that the two tissues (ureteric bud or Wolffian duct and nephrogenic mesenchyme) do not differentiate if isolated, and both have a determinative action on organogenesis. Both play the role of inducer with respect to the other. It would appear that there is some specificity in the inducer activity of the mesonephric duct and the ureteric bud. The association of Wolffian duct tissue with differentiating metanephros results in the differentiation of primarily mesonephric tubules, while explants uniting ureteric bud and differentiating metanephros result in further differentiation of metanephric elements.[36] When metanephros primordia of appropriate age are explanted on the chorioallantoic membrane of 7- to 8-day-old embryos, the explant increases in size, differentiates, and develops into a typical metanephros.

The work of Grobstein[35,37] employing mouse kidney has been concerned with the nature and mode of transmission of the inductive influence to the metanephrogenic mesenchyme. He demonstrated that tissue derived from the ureteric bud has the chemical "inducing" capacity to cause differentiation of mouse metanephrogenic mesenchyme even without direct cytoplasmic contact. The active "inducer" passed through the pores of a filter of limited permeability (less than 1 micron in diameter) that separated the two tissues. The inducing factor appears to be a mucoprotein material secreted by the cells into their immediate environment. The inducer is not restricted to primitive ureteric-bud epithelial tissue. Grobstein found that certain other embryonic epithelial tissues (that is, the neural cord) also induced kidney tubule formation in vitro. Several other in vitro "inducers" with similar inductive specificity have subsequently been described.[38-41]

Further studies have shown that the integrity of embryonic induction can be influenced by metabolites, hormones, vitamins, and various physical or chemical "shocks" which act by altering the interaction of one tissue on another. More knowledge of the specificity of the control mechanisms regulating tissue differentiation and embryonic induction will be needed before we can hope to have an adequate explanation of the basic mechanisms responsible for abnormal structural organogenesis of the kidney. The interested reader can consult the excellent review of Hay.[42]

MORPHOLOGIC CHANGES ASSOCIATED WITH NEPHRON INDUCTION

The first morphologic signs of induction of nephron formation are the condensation of a solid mass of mesenchymal cells in close contact with but distinct from the proliferating tissue of the ampulla forming the growing end of the primitive collecting tubule (Plate 1.1A and B, taken from Oliver). The immediate physical proximity of the future nephron and its collecting duct is established at the time of nephron induction. This direct demonstration by Oliver of the close early relationship makes untenable the theory which attributes the origin of blind-ending nephrons found in polycystic kidneys to the failure of these two simultaneously differentiating parts to "find each other" and unite later in organogenesis.[15] There is no evidence that they are ever spatially independent.

The first evidence of nephronic development appears as a vesicle forms and the central cavity elongates, assuming a tubular form with the appearance of demarcations by surface grooves that mark the site of subsequent development of two elements—one the glomerulus which occupies the most distal part of the growing projection and a globular enlargement between the rudimentary glomerulus and the connecting tubule representing Stoerk's complex (Plate 1.1C). Stoerk's complex elaborates the hairpin loop of Henle and the pars recta of the proximal tubule.[15]

It is of interest that the two ends of the developing nephron, the glomerulus and the connecting tubule, become fixed by attachment soon after the vesicle starts developing into a nephron. The developing glomerulus and Bowman's capsule become fixed as vascularization proceeds and a clearly recognizable glomerular arteriole appears attached to the rudimentary glomerulus (see Plate 1.2A and B). The connecting tubule is already fixed by its attachment to the ampulla of the collecting tubule. The loop of Henle is formed by tangential growth of the tubule forming the bend of Stoerk's complex. It grows along the axis of the kidney, oriented toward the pyramid.

The early vascularization of the glomerulus by ingrowth of mesenchymal vessels can be seen to result in the molding of Bowman's space as a result of growth expansion of the proliferating tuft. The growth of vascular tissue molds the terminal portion of the continuous lumen of the nephron into the glomerular cup. The continuity of Bowman's space in the invaginated crescent-like glomerular anlage with the proximal convolution is evident in Plate 1.3A. The proliferating glomerular tuft and its efferent and afferent arterioles are easily identifiable before the glomerular cup has been fully formed. When it is complete, it covers the glomerular vascular system except for the vascular pole, where the efferent and afferent arterioles enter the Malpighian corpuscle. The continuity of the thick visceral layer of Bowman's capsule and the thin parietal layer can be easily identified.

The development of the unique glomerular arterial supply occurs
pari passu with the development of the general configuration of the arterial system of the adult organ. The glomerular afferent arterioles are
extensions of intralobular branches of arcuate arteries (Plate 1.4). Oliver
found that the adult pattern of arterial blood supply of the kidney was
already evident by the second month of gestation. The general appearance
of the nephrons in various stages of development toward the end of that
month can be appreciated by examining the specimen shown in Plate
1.5, which consists of two collecting trees from one of the calyces of
the kidney at 2½ months. The details of formation of the branches of
the collecting system and of the process responsible for the final arrangement of nephrons and collecting ducts found in the mature kidney are
presented later.

CONTROVERSIAL STAGES IN THE DEVELOPMENT OF THE HUMAN KIDNEY

There is general agreement among embryologists on events up to this
point, but descriptions of the subsequent happenings are quite divergent.
The major points of concern involve: (a) the mechanism whereby continuity is established between nephrons and collecting ducts; (b) formation of the glomerulus; and (c) the mechanism responsible for segregation of the nephrons to the cortex and branches of the collecting tree
to the medulla. Each of these aspects will be discussed in some detail
since they form the basis for hypotheses as to the causes of renal dysplasia
and polycystic changes. The review of the traditional theories is timely
in light of recent morphologic studies employing microdissection and
electron microscopy that have greatly increased the amount of quantitative information available on the developmental anatomy of the human
kidney.

I have condensed some of the many aspects Oliver covers in his monograph *Nephrons and Kidneys*,[1] choosing for emphasis some of the major
events of differentiation that underlie the complex structural organization
achieved in the mature kidney. Some of the areas of controversy are
exposed but no attempt has been made to present a complete "airing
of divergence" on this broad subject. The reader who seeks more detailed
information is advised to read Oliver's monograph, where a complete
treatment is provocatively presented.

The Mechanism whereby Continuity is Established between Nephrons and Collecting Ducts

In the traditional view[15] the newly formed renal vesicle elongates and enlarges to form the various parts of the nephron; at a still later time, the distal end of the nephronic tubule establishes contact with the distal end of the collecting tubule, then a continuous lumen between the parts is formed in some undescribed manner. In the mature nephron continuity between the nephron and its collecting tubule is established by that portion anatomically labeled by Oliver the *connecting tubule*.

The precise limits of the *connecting tubule* in earlier descriptions were impossible to establish histologically and the exact embryonic origin is still uncertain. The term is used to describe that portion of the nephron distal to the distal convoluted tubule after its emergence from the "nephronic packet" (the glomerulus and its two convoluted tubules). It differs in histologic characteristics from the distal convolution and may join it to the collecting duct by way of an arcade. Oliver has demonstrated by the use of microdissection that it arises from the nephronic tubule. It can be identified in the earliest stage of nephron formation lying in close proximity to its induced renal vesicle and is frequently the first segment of the newly forming nephron to become histologically recognizable with differentiation.

The demonstration that the *connecting tubule* is an integral part of the nephron is not to be viewed as a minor taxonomic accomplishment, since Oliver states that "without its recognition a rational concept of renal architectonics is impossible."[43] He attributes much of the final spatial arrangement of nephrons in the mature kidney to its unique proliferative proclivity. It may be short or so long that it equals the rest of the nephron in volume and length.

The bioengineering of the process of fusion and lumen formation at the point of insertion is demonstrably accomplished by cellular rearrangement, as shown in Plate 1.6A and B. Disturbances in this phenomenon could result in obstruction of nephrons and localized cystic dilatation involving secondarily segments of the collecting-duct system. The development of cystic lesions of *connecting tubules* or distal convolutions could occur in widely varied areas of the kidney, however, because of the variability of the length and location of this connecting segment in nephrons in different layers of the fully differentiated cortex. These observations cast doubt on the validity of attempts at classification of types of polycystic disease as cortical or medullary or nephronic or collecting duct on the sole basis of the observed location of cystic cavities in different levels of the fully developed cortex or medulla.

Formation of the Glomerulus

The earliest concept of the development of the glomerulus was an attempt to explain how it achieved the structure seen in the adult. Bowman[44] defined its structure in 1842 as a network of capillaries set in the end of the renal tubule. Early observers are quoted by Herring[45] as believing that the glomerulus was formed at the blind hollow end by proliferating capillaries arising from mesenchymal interstitium. By this process (invagination by a proliferating, preformed capillary plexus) the covering of the capillaries within Bowman's capsule by the epithelial membrane representing the invaginated (visceral) layer of the epithelium of the blind end of the tubule was explained.

The invagination theory was not, however, unanimously accepted. Herring's direct observations on glomerulogenesis did not offer support for this simplified concept. He reported that the glomerulus develops by ingrowth of solid cords of primitive endothelial cells into the adjacent still-solid vesicle formed by the mass of primitive tubular cells. It is only after the two cell groups intermingle that the first evidence of a capsular space develops by a splitting apart or delamination of the plaque. The resulting slit-like space then enlarges to surround the intermingled mass of endothelial and epithelial cells. Herring indicated that there was no direct evidence to support the existence of a process implied by the invagination theory of a preformed hollow Malpighian corpuscle being indented by preformed growing capillaries.

Further indirect support for the invagination theory arose as a result of the attention given by pathologists to the work of Zimmermann[46] and von Möllendorff.[47] The characteristic structure of the adult glomerulus was ascribed by them to a developmental process involving the invagination of a hollow vesicle by the capillaries. The network of capillary loops found in the adult glomerulus was pictured as being situated in a "sling" made up of the invaginated basement membrane and cells of the Malpighian corpuscle. The term mesangium was applied to this sling-like structure. It included fibroblast-like cells and connective tissue fibers along with endothelial cells, which lined the lumen of the capillaries.[48]

Although dispute continued, the general mesangial or sling concept (with its developmental implication that the invagination concept was correct) was generally accepted until the application of electron microscopy to the study of glomerulogenesis in the rat by Hall[49] and in the human kidney by Kurtz.[50] The direct observations of these investigators confirmed the earlier view proposed by Herring[45] and provided no evidence to support the view of a hollow vesicle indented by preformed capillaries. Their data can be summarized as having shown that the vesicular space is altered by differential epithelial growth in one area with infolding to form the layer comprising the visceral layer of Bowman's capsule internally and the glomerular cleft seen externally.

The invagination of the lateral wall of the elongating vesicle has been demonstrated by Oliver[1] to involve growth transformation resulting from physical changes caused by the proliferating epithelial cells of the vesicle. The glomerular cleft (Plate 1.2) delineates the location of the future glomerular tuft. The subsequent growth of endothelial anlage from pre-existing vascular tissue in the interstitial mesenchyme into this cleft has now been well described.[50-53] It is apparent that it was an oversimplification to assume that the wall of the end of the renal tubule of the primitive nephron was mechanically invaginated by penetrating growth of preformed capillaries. Invagination of the primitive vesicle is a de novo growth process involved in the development of the glomerular tuft.

Lewis[52] has presented convincing evidence that the vascular tissue of the metanephros enters the cleft in the developing vesicle to form the capillaries of the glomerular tuft. He employed injection of the vascular system of the developing kidney with colloidal dye and microdissection to clarify the origin of the glomerular capillaries. The question of an in situ origin for the glomerular capillaries[54,55] seems pedantic since all of the blood vessels of the kidney arise in situ after initial growth of the renal artery and vein at the hilus. Renal vascularization is accomplished by progressively advancing transformation of both intertubular and intraglomerular mesenchymal vascular spaces in a process associated with conversion of a sinusoidal plexus to a capillary configuration. Lewis found that vascularization of the glomerular tuft is a concomitant part of vascularization in situ of the kidney as a whole and should not be considered an independent event in glomerular development unrelated to phenomena occurring in closely adjacent epithelial and mesenchymal cells in the differentiating metanephros.

Arterial channels were observed to develop by arborization through the sinusoidal plexus of branches of the renal artery. This process has been confirmed by the use of similar techniques by Osathanondh and Potter[56] and in greater microscopic detail by Aoki.[53] Lewis concludes that "whatever the mechanism the cortical plexus is remodeled to produce arterial channels leading to the glomeruli."

A diagrammatic representation from Lewis is reproduced as Fig. 1.7, because it best illustrates the manner in which the developing glomeruli are vascularized while arterial and venous vascularization of the kidney occurs pari passu. The actual early arterial pattern at 2½ months of fetal life is also shown in Plate 1.5. The efferent and afferent arterioles of the glomerulus make their appearance as the capillaries of the glomerulus become enclosed in the spherical glomerular capsule.

The next question concerns the exact manner of embryologic formation of the filtering membrane of the glomerulus, which is still a matter of debate. The ultrastructure of the mature filtration membrane has been described in minute detail in current texts[57,58] and it is assumed that the reader will consult them for familiarity with this aspect of the subject.

It was noted by Kurtz[50] that the earliest evidence of basement membrane structure (lamina densa) consisted in a thin, slightly dense band seen primarily at points of apposition between epithelial and endothelial cells. This suggests that the primitive membrane originated from interaction of epithelial and endothelial cells. It was also noted that the immediate presence of epithelial cell processes was necessary for completing the differentiation of the endothelial cell mass, for only in such areas did the endothelial cells present a mature appearance.

Kurtz has shown that differentiation of the mature glomerular membrane first involves the formation of two separate linings—the internal endothelium and the external epithelium (podocytes)—which make a "sandwich" between which appears the discrete and continuous glomerular basement membrane that forms the actual definitive filter of the glomerulus. The formation of the glomerular basement membrane thus involves both epithelial and endothelial cell activity, as does the maintenance of physiologic integrity during its functional life.

These findings advance the concept that a dependent and possibly inductive relationship may be established between the epithelial cells forming Bowman's capsule and the mesenchymal cells arising from the interstitial vascular system that penetrate after invagination of the vesicle begins. Aoki[53] cites considerable indirect evidence supporting the view that the glomerular basement membrane arises by a process of tissue interaction that appears analogous to the embryonic induction responsible for the initial differentiation of the metanephros. When the renal vascular system is not available as in vitro culture of explants[59] or experi-

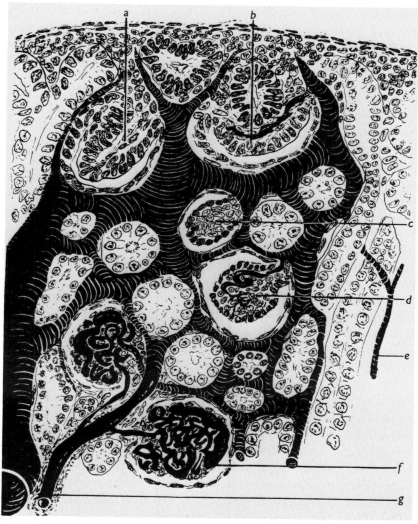

FIGURE 1.7 A diagram of the thickness of the cortex of a developing injected kidney, showing the manner in which the glomeruli are vascularized. *a*—a very early glomerulus, not vascularized. *b*—a similar glomerulus containing a strand of dye continuous with surrounding sinusoids. *c*—a medium-age glomerulus, dense and unvascularized. *d*—commencing vascularization of a glomerulus. *e*—vasa recta entering medullary ray from sinusoidal plexus. *f*—well-vascularized glomerulus. *g*—artery elaborating from the cortical plexus and lying beside a large vein draining the plexus. (From O. J. Lewis.[52])

mental induction of isolated metanephrogenic blastema,[37] there is no formation of glomerular corpuscles; only tubules develop. The development
of rudimentary to fully mature glomeruli has, however, been observed
when fragments of embryonic kidney have been explanted into vascularized organs.[36,60] If these observations can be confirmed it would resolve
the controversy, since it is generally agreed that development of the
glomerulus requires participation of the interstitial vascular system in
some manner.

In Aoki's view[58] the interstitial tissue that migrates into the cleft of
the renal vesicle differentiates into two types of cells found in the mature
glomerulus, the endothelial cell of the capillary wall and the mesangial
cell. He found no evidence to support in situ development of erythrocytes.
This observation gains support from the findings of Vernier and Birch-
Andersen[61] in their studies of the circulation of the glomerulus in the
developing human kidney (using injection of contrast material via the
umbilical artery in specimens obtained from early abortion). These researchers failed to detect any capillary containing erythrocytes not intermixed with injected particles of ferritin or carbon, and the ferritin particles appeared in capillaries of all but the most immature glomeruli
via anastomosis of developing tuft vessels with the arterial system.

The process of histogenesis producing the three components of the
mature glomerular filtering membrane may be biochemically comparable
to that produced experimentally by McLoughlin[62] through contact of
epithelial and connective tissue. It is possible that the large increase in
endothelial surface and dilatation in capillary lumina and stretching of
epithelial cytoplasmic processes characteristic of the glomerular filter is
produced by increasing hydrostatic pressure that arises as circulation increases in the proliferating capillaries growing into the glomerular tuft.

The permeability characteristics of the basement membrane of the
differentiated glomerulus in the human fetus have not been extensively
studied. They were investigated by Vernier and Birch-Andersen,[61] who
found that the fetal glomerular capillary appeared to be more permeable
than the mature membrane. The glomerular basement membrane is
thinner at birth (1,000 Å) than in the adult (2,500 Å), not achieving
adult width until about three years of age.[63]

The Mechanism Responsible for Segregation of Nephrons to the Cortex

The growth process that accounts for the segregation of all nephrons
to the cortex and collecting ducts to the medulla in the mature kidney

has not been defined in detail. The observed radial branching of the growing primitive ureteric bud adequately accounts for the formation of divisions of the major and minor calyces and the major units comprising the collecting trees that arise from the ducts of Bellini. The problem arises when one attempts to account for the final appearance of the collecting system where all of the early generations of collecting tubules produced by ureteric bud divisions are found to be bare of nephrons.

The first formed nephrons attached to the collecting ducts observed in Oliver's study seemed to have moved their attachment to collecting ducts produced at a later time and to be moving toward the outer portion (cortex) of the developing fetal kidney. Oliver found nephrons to be present on the VIIth and VIIIth generation of collecting ducts when examined at an early stage (2⅛ months, see Plate 1.7), while there were no nephrons found attached to these generations of collecting ducts on an older specimen from a 2½-month fetus (Plate 1.5). This could be explained by postulating a differential growth process whereby nephrons develop fully only after several divisions of the collecting system have already been formed, or by assuming that induced nephrons can detach themselves and migrate freely before establishing their definitive attachment to collecting tubules. Neither view is supported by available data.

A corollary of the first view is that the earliest nephrons formed degenerate and do so in an involutional process analogous to that occurring in the pronephros and mesonephros. Degeneration of induced nephrons associated with the primary and secondary generations of collecting tubules was proposed by Kampmeier[64] to explain the segregation in the mature kidney of nephrons to the cortex and major branches of the collecting tree to the medulla. As a consequence of the lack of agreement about the growth mechanism involved, since some explanation is necessary to account for final renal architectural form, selective nephron survival in the developing metanephros has been widely accepted as a normal growth process of renal organogenesis. Disturbances in this process have been proposed as a mechanism (dysgenesis) to account for some cystic changes that occur,[45,58,64] such as incomplete degeneration that leads to blockage of the tubular lumen before cessation of glomerular function, resulting in cyst formation.

Oliver points out that Kampmeier in his study of complete serial sections of twenty-three fetal kidneys 6 weeks to 5 months of age reported the average number of degenerating nephrons found per kidney was less than five.[65] Oliver found no numerically significant degeneration of nephrons in his dissection at any period of renal development, a conclusion in agreement with the findings of Huber,[66] Felix,[15] and Peter[14] in their studies of histologic sections which were directed specifically toward the discovery of such a possible involutionary change predominating in the pronephros and mesonephros. Oliver concluded that while destruction of nephrons undoubtedly occurs as the first six of the ultimate fifteen generations of the collecting system expand to form the pelvis, "this cannot play a very great part in the evolution of the architectural pattern of the million nephrons constituting the definitive kidney."[65]

The occurrence of glomerular degeneration in occasional glomeruli has been noted by all pathologists who have examined the normal fetal and postnatal kidney. This process involves single nephrons in scattered areas of the cortex and results in complete fibrosis of the affected glomerulus and atrophy of the arteriolar-glomerular unit, so-called congenital glomerulosclerosis. Ljungqvist[67] did not find any degenerating glomeruli in specimens younger than 7 months of gestation. He found that this process becomes evident in the last trimester (seventh to ninth month of uterine life) and continues for the first two years of life. The process, however, does not play a significant role in renal development in the quantitative sense.

Ljungqvist was especially interested in the mechanism of the fetal and postnatal development of the intrarenal arterial pattern. He reported finding evidence (using microangiography and microdissection) of another process of glomerular degeneration that involved some of the nephrons in the pelvic and periarcuate region of the developing kidney. The degeneration of their glomerular vessels was associated with persistence of their arteriolar vessels via direct communication of the afferent and efferent glomerular arteriole to form arteriolae rectae verae penetrating into the medulla without passing through a glomerular capillary plexus. He has proposed this as a mechanism that operates postnatally and even into adulthood to produce the unique intrarenal blood-flow pattern found in the juxtamedullary regions of the mature kidney.

There is no evidence to support the hypothesis that selective degeneration of the first metanephric nephrons formed occurs because they are primitive in the sense of being similar to the tubules of the mesonephros. The two sorts of nephrons have a different phylogenetic and ontogenetic history. The uriniferous tubules of the mesonephros form separately from the collecting system (mesonephric duct), which arises from a process of fusion of the ends of the pronephric tubules. The sequence in the metanephros is reversed, since duct development precedes the appearance of nephrons. Oliver has demonstrated histologically recognizable metanephric nephrons joined to patent collecting ducts in the youngest specimen (8 to 9 weeks of gestation) he examined (Plate 1.7).

More direct evidence is provided by the demonstration of functional differences between chick mesonephric and human metanephric tubules by Cameron and Chambers.[68] These workers provided the first direct evidence (in vitro) that human embryonic proximal tubules function (that is, they are able to actively transport dyestuffs) at least at 3½ months of age. They observed that the proximal tubules of the human metanephros maintained a lower pH in tubular fluid (pH 7.0) than in the culture medium (7.4 to 7.6), in contrast to conditions in the chick mesonephros where the pH of the tubular fluid always approximated that of the surrounding medium.

The movement of nephrons to the cortex and the final attachment of most of their connecting tubules to the last few generations of collecting ducts formed could be accounted for by assuming that there are differential rates of growth of certain portions in the proliferating buds of the dividing collecting tubules that account for the apparent change of attachment. This mechanism is known as Peter's transport hypothesis.

Peter's transport hypothesis[14] proposes that accelerated interstitial growth of the tubule occurs in localized intercalated zones below the place of attachment of the induced nephrons which are growing in close proximity to the ampulla of the tubule. By this mechanism the newly formed nephrons are carried forward with the tip of the dividing collecting tubule and its ampulla, and in this process the older nephrons can accumulate on the advancing tip. The new-formed vesicles appear on the outside of the links of the division of the tubule and not within the fork. The initial nephrons induced on the ampulla by the early generation of dividing collecting tubules are carried forward with the proliferating (dividing) portion of the ampulla because of the more active growth of the immediately adjacent lower intercalated portion of the recently divided collecting tubule (see Fig. 1.8).

Oliver has demonstrated such broadened localized zones of accelerated growth in dissected specimens which have been specially stained to show details of proliferating cellular growth (see Plate 1.3B). The ultimate partition of nephrons among the advancing ampullae cannot produce an even distribution, for after each division of the tubule the ampulla

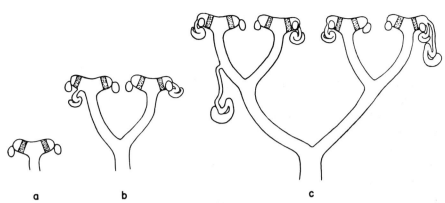

a   b   c

FIGURE 1.8 Peter's diagram, showing his hypothetical intercalated zone of localized accelerated interstitial growth (dotted area) which carries the nephrons forward with the extending and dividing collecting tubules. To the left in *b* and *c* he shows one nephron which has been left behind; such a possibility must be admitted, but none was found in Oliver's dissections. At the extreme right in *c* his concept of the origin of an arcade is shown. (From K. Peter.[14])

inducing a new nephron on one branch will have carried along one or more nephrons from the previous bifurcation while the ampulla on the other branch of the latest division will have received none. This is evident in Figs. 1.8 and 1.9. If all of the nephrons which are induced upon the successively dividing collecting ducts (the closed divided portion) are transported to the cortex of the kidney by Peter's transport mechanism, the end result would have certain quantitative results and spatial relations that should be demonstrable in the mature cortex.

Oliver's studies have provided direct evidence of the frequency distribution of the various patterns of nephronic accumulation (1–2, 1–3, 1–4, and so forth) on pairs of terminal dividing ducts that would be predicted from the forward march of nephrons diagrammed in the abacus of Fig. 1.9. The "forward march" involves only those nephrons formed during the creation of the closed divided portion of the collecting trees. It represents the initial step in the establishment of cortex and medulla by separation of ducts and nephrons. In the final stage of nephron formation the ducts cease to divide but continue to grow through the depth of the thickening cortex, forming the open system and inducing more nephrons until they cease growing beneath the capsule. In the final kidney this descriptive distinction between the open and closed portions of the collecting system can no longer be recognized.

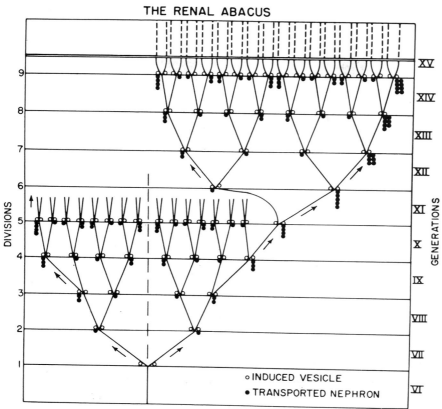

FIGURE 1.9 Graphic presentation of the structural and quantitative results of Peter's transport mechanism resulting in the accumulation of nephrons on late generations of the collecting ducts. (From J. Oliver.[1])

The maturing interstitial growth so modifies the latter generation that it blends both portions into the definitive cortex of the adult kidney. The nephrons involved in the transport process form the lowermost nephrons which lie in the juxtamedullary zone of the cortex.

Induction of new nephrons would be associated with displacement of the connecting tubule of the already attached earlier nephrons (now more mature), yet maintain their continuity with the connecting tubule of the newly induced nephrons. Thus this transport process also results in arcade formation. Arcades consist of a string of nephrons joined serially by connecting tubules that fuse and ultimately enter a single collecting duct. This process explains how the first-formed nephrons transported to the periphery of the collecting system have a means of connecting these deep-lying nephrons by the arcades to a collecting system which will in a sense overgrow them, because the top of the medullary ray in the adult kidney is several millimeters beyond the region where the corticomedullary nephrons lie.

Oliver points out that current descriptions of renal development which have tacitly accepted Peter's general hypothesis of forward movement of nephrons ignore the quantitative necessities of the consequences of such a process. The forward movement is seen as a mechanism accounting for the movement of the nephrons induced on early generations of collecting ducts to the cortex, thus clearing some of the collecting ducts of nephron attachments, but the induction of nephrons and formation of collecting-duct branches is viewed as a random process. This view cannot account for the structural uniformity of the end result, a kidney composed of approximately 1,000,000 nephrons.

Oliver's careful studies provide direct evidence in support of the view that the shifting of nephrons occurs in an orderly manner, as does their induction. The induction of one nephron on the lateral aspect of each ampulla formed by the dividing collecting duct is the only process that is entirely consistent with the pattern he found of new and accumulating older nephrons on various generations of the collecting ducts at the early as well as the final stage of development of the kidney. Two quotations from page 15 of the Oliver book[1] put the case for a regulated process most effectively:

If two nephrons formed on both sides of the ampulla on both limbs of each division or randomly about it, there would result more nephrons than are present in the final kidney.

It might be supposed that with such an active increase in nephrons as is observed in the first months there would occur a considerable accumulation of them on the terminal ampullae. But since the ducts themselves are dividing, a consideration of the two series of geometrical progression, one describing 9 dichotomous divisions of the tubule (2^n, or 2, 4, 8, 16 . . . 512) and the other the induction of 2 nephrons, one on the lateral side of each limb of each of the divisions ($2\,[2^n] - 2$, or 2, 6, 14, 30 . . . 1,022) shows that the number of nephrons which can accumulate on each of the terminal divisions is remarkably small, approaching 2 as a limit, *providing* all nephrons were evenly distributed among them.

The spatial relations of the patterns formed with successive tubular division and nephron induction that were found by Oliver are consistent with Peter's transport mechanism and make it clear that there cannot be an even distribution of nephrons among the advancing ampullae of the growing ducts. Appreciation of this complex process will be greatly aided by the graphic representation of this transformation that is provided from Oliver (again on page 15) along with his eloquent comments:

> To adequately describe or to comprehend any textual description of the detail of this forward march of the individual nephrons and their resulting deployment in accumulated groupings which change with each step of the advance would require the mental facilities of blind-fold chess. A graphic presentation has therefore been prepared in the form of what can be called a renal abacus [Fig. 9]. This figure is not a diagram representing the development of renal structures, but only a graphic framework on which, as the name indicates, the reader can visualize, follow, and sum up in quantitative terms the movement of added units as they are transported along a series of dividing paths.

Rigorous examination and quantitative comparison of the agreement and discordance between this hypothetical process and the configurations and actual patterns found in dissection is available in Oliver's work. The accumulation of several nephrons on one collecting duct is an important first step in formation of the arcades that drain the deeper nephrons of the cortex.

While some nephrons produced by the earliest generations of collecting ducts may be lost, the actual number involved would be inconsequential to the final number of nephrons formed. Only the nephrons produced by the first five generations of collecting-duct divisions are subject to degeneration if Peter's transport hypothesis is invoked to account for movement of the subsequently formed nephrons to the cortex. Since the process of duct division is largely dichotomous, there is a geometric progression in the number of nephrons produced with each successive division of collecting ducts. The great majority of nephrons found in the adult kidney (about three-fourths) consequently will arise from the last two generations of collecting ducts (XIV and XV), and approximately half of these from the last generation.

The theoretic estimate of nephrons resulting from this architectonic theory is in close agreement with the estimate of total nephrons in the adult kidney based on the mean values found by Oliver in actual dissection of complete collecting trees and their attached nephrons.[69] The observed distribution was 615,897 nephrons contributed by the XIVth generation of collecting systems and 550,202 nephrons by the XVth generation. Oliver's direct observations by actual dissection support both propositions (Peter's transport hypothesis and dichotomous division of the collecting ducts). The period of degeneration of nephrons involves the first two months of renal development and is limited to the area where spatial relations are unique because it is the site of transformation of the first generations of the collecting tubules into the major and minor calyces.

FORMATION OF THE COLLECTING SYSTEM

The collecting trees of the mature kidney drain into minor calyces that in turn empty into the major calyces and pelvis and ureter. The minor and major calyces of the mature kidney are derived from the first few (Ist to Vth) divisions of the ureteric bud. The duct divisions not incorporated into the pelvocalyceal complex disappear, as do all of the attached nephrons. Oliver found that the VIth division of the ureteric bud was the first division after which all of the duct divisions that formed (assuming dichotomous division to be the normal process) persisted and could be accounted for by dissection of the developing kidney. He has documented the stages in the development of the mature collecting-duct system by examining primitive calyces and their branches of the dividing ductal system from kidneys in early fetal life (2⅛ months) to term.

A primitive calyx and its provisional ducts from the earliest specimen examined is shown in Plate 1.7. The nephrons in this specimen are attached to ducts which are only two later divisions than the calyx (VI). The widening of the cavity of the calyx with growth by obliterating some of the primitive duct space to include within the calyx the early generations of the primitive ducts is shown in a slightly older specimen (2½ months) in Plate 1.5, in which two complete primitive collecting trees have been preserved along with the most terminal branchings and their attached nephrons.

The successive changes that occur in the further branching of the collecting-tree units are evident in the specimens at 3¾ months (Plate 1.8) and 5 months (Plate 1.9). The arabic numbers designate divisions of the collecting ducts subsequent to that forming the minor calyx (VI) and the roman numerals designate the generations descending from the first division of the ureteric bud designated as I. Oliver has found that only the last few generations of the collecting ducts (XIII to XV) have attached nephrons in the mature kidney. The explanation of how all of the nephrons formed on earlier divisions could move to this cortical position and leave the intermediate branches of the collecting tree (VI to XII) devoid of nephrons has been discussed above.

In the mature kidney each major collecting-tree unit has its origin at a single duct of Bellini which empties into a minor calyx through the renal papillae in the area cribrosa. The ideal architectonic pattern of the collecting system can be visualized as successive multiple branching units beginning with the VIth division and including the last division of the primitive ureteric duct (XV) that produces the final generation of collecting ducts extending into the cortex. The chronology of this process can be emphasized by citing three developmental landmarks:

(1) The initial appearance of the primitive ureteric bud is at about the fifth week of gestation (Fig. 1.5) and division occurs shortly thereafter.

(2) The first six divisions of the ureteric bud have taken place by the eighth to ninth week.

(3) The last division (XVth) is completed by the fifth month (Plate 1.9).

With the last division the formation of that portion of the *collecting tree* that Oliver calls the *closed portion* is accomplished. The further growth of these terminal ducts forms the open *cortical collecting system,* which Oliver designates as including all the subsequent branches of a single collecting tubule from its entrance into the cortex to its termination beneath the surface of the kidney, along with all the connecting tubules of the attached nephrons. Though subsequent growth of the proliferating collecting tubules occurs without further division, nephron induction still continues actively as these terminal divisions of the collecting system extend to reach the outermost part of the cortex.

The great variation in length of collecting-tubule segments can be accounted for by variations in the rate of linear growth of the different generations of collecting ducts. Some grow more rapidly than others, producing long stretches of branchless segments in the medulla alternating with short segments. The linear growth of the collecting system determines the distance from the area cribrosa in the papilla to the cortical capsule. The configuration of the outer medulla in the adult kidney reflects these different rates of growth during fetal life when one or more of several generations of collecting ducts grew at the expense of the others.

Oliver distinguishes three regions in the collecting system where characteristically differing rates of growth are discernible during early renal development: (1) the cortical area, including the XIVth and XVth generations; (2) a central medullary region composed of generations XI, XII, and XIII; and (3) an internal medullary zone, including the papilla and generations VI to X. Growth of the collecting system in the central medullary region is at a maximum from the fourth month to term. During this period there is a marked lag in growth of the cortical and internal medullary areas. At about the seventh month of fetal life there is a wave of accelerated medullary growth at the level of the XIth generation of collecting ducts, which spreads throughout higher generations (Xth to XVth) of the system to include ultimately the terminal collecting ducts after birth. The almost complete absence of growth after birth in the first generations of the collecting system and internal and central medullary region is in marked contrast to this accelerated growth seen throughout the outer medulla and cortex and accounts for the anatomic similarity of the papillary area in the infant and adult kidney.

QUANTITATIVE RELATIONS BETWEEN NEPHRONS AND CORTICAL COLLECTING SYSTEMS IN THE ADULT KIDNEY

Oliver's studies involving direct counts to determine the total number of collecting-duct systems in the normal adult kidney have revealed striking numerical agreement between quantitative estimates based on (1) direct observation of the total number of branches and divisions present in the average collecting system, (2) the mean number of total nephrons in the adult kidney, and (3) the theoretic expectations derived by his architectonic description. These observations provide the basis for his theory that the development of the cortical collecting-duct system and the total number of attached nephrons in the kidney are not the result of random growth and transformation. He has elaborated an arithmetical concept[70] that could be considered as analogous to "programmed" kidney growth. It accounts for the kidney's characteristic medullary and cortical structure and the mean complement of 1,209,000 nephrons (range 810,000 to 1,780,000) found by direct counts on kidneys of children and adults by Moberg.[71]

The formulation of this concept required the development of an arithmetical scheme that could account for the architectural pattern of the medulla and cortex and the number of duct divisions and nephrons found in the mature kidney from 2½ months of fetal life up to adulthood. In order to understand the concept of regulated renal development, familiarity with Oliver's nomenclature is essential. It is given in Table 1.1, along with the ideal form of collecting-tree formation.

The number of ultimate divisions arising from the primitive ureteric bud is indicated by roman numerals (I to XV). Each new group of collecting ducts formed by successive duct division is defined as a generation and identified specifically by roman numerals denoting the duct divisions that account for its production after the first division (I) formed by the ureteric bud. The average number of ducts of Bellini entering one papilla in the human kidney is about forty.[10] Assuming dichotomous division to be the usual pattern of production of new ductules, the total number of collecting ducts found in the adult kidney can be accounted for by assuming that the VIth division of the progeny of the primitive ureteric bud is represented by the ducts of Bellini and is the first generation of collecting tubules whose progeny (duct divisions and formed nephrons) will persist throughout all of the remaining stages of renal development. If ideal conditions are assumed to prevail, nine subsequent divisions (VII to XV) of the collecting ducts would result in a minimum of 1,023 generations of collecting ducts in each tree and a minimum total of 360,000 ducts comprising the whole collecting system found in each adult kidney.

On the basis of Oliver's detailed determination of the number and order of divisions of the collecting ducts forming the closed medullary collecting system and the open cortical system, and employing Peter's transport mechanism to account for the finding that only the last three generations of collecting ducts are nephron-bearing in the definitive kidney, it becomes possible to compare the validity of his architectonic theory of a programmed process or ordered duct division, nephron induction, and nephron transport with the number of collecting-duct systems and nephrons found in the average kidney. No previous embryologic or mor-

TABLE 1.1 Nomenclature and arithmetical relations of divisions and generations (from J. Oliver[1])

Generations I to V (taken up into pelvis)	Number of generations in —	
	each collecting tree	average kidney with 44 pores and 8 papillae = 352 collecting trees
1st persisting VIth generation	1	352
1st division followed by VIIth generation	2	704
2nd division followed by VIIIth generation	4	1,408
3rd division followed by IXth generation	8	2,816
4th division followed by Xth generation	16	5,632
5th division followed by XIth generation	32	11,264
6th division followed by XIIth generation	64	22,528
7th division followed by XIIIth generation	128	45,056
8th division followed by XIVth generation	256	90,112
9th[a] division followed by XVth generation	512 or total of >1,023	180,224 or total of >360,096[b]

[a] About 38 percent of the ducts do not divide nine times.

[b] Of these only the XIIIth to XVth generations (315,392) bear nephrons in the definitive kidney.

phologic description has proposed an explanation consistent with such an eventuality.

Actual dissection by Oliver has revealed that not all of the collecting ducts divide a ninth time (38 percent do not, as indicated in Table 1.1) and only the XIIIth to XVth generations are nephron-bearing in the adult kidney. There is some variability among collecting systems. Oliver has determined the distribution of different types of cortical tree systems that are nephron-bearing and the mean number of nephrons on each type of cortical system. The XVth generation drained more nephrons as a rule than the XIVth, and even fewer nephrons were found on the XIIIth generation which lies lowermost in the cortex. He has used the data he obtained from dissections of a series of five kidneys to calculate the total number of nephron-bearing ducts and nephrons in the kidney with the following result:

XVth generation of the collecting
system would contribute $152,834 \times 3.6^* =$ 550,202 nephrons
XIVth generation of the collecting
system would contribute $136,866 \times 4.5\ =$ 615,897 nephrons
XIIIth generation of the collecting
system would contribute $22,811 \times 2.8\ =$ 63,871 nephrons
    TOTAL   312,511   1,229,970 nephrons

A comparison of these results with the theoretic ideal shown in Table 1.1 shows that the agreement between calculated and observed counts of total collecting ducts is sufficiently close to offer strong support to the validity of Oliver's developmental description as an explanation for ordered development regulating the number of collecting ducts and nephrons in the definitive kidney.

THE KIDNEY LATER IN GESTATION

At the Fifth Month

By the fifth month of gestation the configurational irregularities seen in the first months in the collecting system and the developing nephrons have disappeared. Considerable maturation of the medullary collecting-tree systems has now occurred. All of the nephrons have moved to the periphery and the demarcation of the cortex and medulla is readily apparent, as seen in Plate 1.9. The kidney, however, still contains only about a third of the nephrons that will ultimately be formed. The extensions of the terminal collecting ducts will grow toward the cortex in the form of spear-like tips without further division to form the *open direct portion* of the collecting system. The nephrons of the lower cortical region were the earliest formed and together with the *closed divided portion* of the collecting system occupy the juxtamedullary zone and deeper portions of the definitive cortex. Differential rates of growth have already resulted in the spatial orientation of medullary and cortical struc-

---

* Mean number of nephrons per system.

tures that anticipates the final configuration of the mature kidney. The cellular differentiation of the older nephrons has progressed so that proximal and distal coiled convolutions and loops of Henle with thin and thick portions are clearly delineated.

During the Fifth to Ninth Months

By the end of the fourth month the final XV generations of the collecting-duct system have been formed by nine more divisions of the ducts after the VIth division. The ducts produced in the first six divisions have been modeled into the pelvocalycine system. The *closed divided portion* of the collecting-duct system and all of its branches have now been formed. Growth of the ducts will still occur to develop the spatial relationships found in the mature kidney. The growth of the *closed divided portion* of the collecting system has up to now been greatest in the midmedullary region.

The growth of the collecting system is at maximum in the outer medullary region during this period while there is a marked lag in growth in the inner (papillary) medullary areas. Postnatal growth will be associated with a further increase in relative rates of growth in cortical as well as outer medullary areas, whereas the larger ducts in the papillary region will increase only slightly in length from birth to 20 years. Active growth deeper into the medulla will alter spatial relations of the portions of nephrons which lie in the medulla (the terminal medullary portion of the pars recta of the proximal convolutions and the loop of Henle).

This fetal period is the one in which cortical growth is most active. New nephrons continue to be formed to complete the normal complement, since only about one-third have previously been formed in the development of the *closed divided portion* of the collecting system. The process of their formation changes, however, and nephronic induction now takes place on the tapering protrusions of the growing ends of the terminal projections of the collecting tubules. These growing ducts comprise what Oliver calls the *open direct portion* of the collecting cortical system. While the induction is similar to that previously described, their *orientation* to the extending ducts that will comprise the terminal cortical collecting system is entirely different. As the vesicles differentiate, the single collecting tubule grows past the point of nephronic attachment with the result that nephrons are distributed separately and in alternating series along the side of the growing tubule. As a consequence, no fusion of their connecting tubules can occur and no arcades form; this accounts for the pattern of the adult kidney in which arcades are limited to the lowest level of the cortex.

Up to the fifth month of gestation the ampullar ends of the dividing collecting ducts have been the inducers of nephron formation and the site where nephrons accumulate. Attachments formed with more than one individual nephron have produced arcades that allow for drainage of the deeper nephrons in the cortex. The distal portions of nephrons forming these arcades join to form an intermediary stretch of tubule which Oliver calls the *connecting tubule* and which joins the nephrons to the collecting-duct system. After the XVth generation of the collecting ducts has appeared, they no longer divide. The new nephrons now formed as the terminal projections of the collecting ducts grow into the cortex are joined individually in alternating patterns along the sides of the growing collecting tubules. Growth of the terminal collecting ducts ends when they reach the capsule with the final induction of two or rarely three nephrons to form the spray (Y) form characteristic of the termination of the mature cortical collecting tubule.

The induction of new nephrons continues until the eighth to ninth month of fetal life. This process normally ceases prior to birth with such regularity that persistence of nephron induction as indicated by finding nephrogenic zones in the subcapsular area was shown by Potter and Thierstein[72] to be a reliable index to gestational age. Macdonald and Emery[73] have confirmed and extended Potter and Thierstein's data, showing that primitive glomeruli are only occasionally seen after the thirty-sixth week of gestation.

It is of interest that the size of the kidney increases most rapidly in the last trimester, as does fetal body weight. This period of growth accounts for 80 to 90 percent of the renal mass present at birth. The weight of the two kidneys at the fifth month is about 2.5 to 3.5 grams, while at term it is normally 20 to 40 grams. As has been pointed out elsewhere, the majority of nephrons found in the mature kidney are produced between the fifth and ninth months. Since the closed portion of the collecting system has already been completed by the fifth month, factors inhibiting cell division and growth after this time would not produce abnormalities in the gross medullary configuration or number of branches of the collecting ducts forming the collecting system. Inhibition of the growth of the open portion could, however, still interfere quantitatively with total nephron formation in a significant manner, since about two-thirds of the total nephrons found in the mature kidney are now being formed.

It should be readily apparent that the opportunity for factors inhibiting cell division in utero to interfere quantitatively with renal organogenesis is still considerable in the last four months of pregnancy. Interference with cell division during this period could still have profound effects by reducing nephron numbers. Such growth inhibition in late gestation may be a factor in those cases of unexplained small-sized kidneys whose structures are grossly normal-appearing (so-called hypoplastic kidneys). This possibility can be investigated experimentally.

RELATIONS BETWEEN CELLULAR DIFFERENTIATION AND MORPHOLOGIC AND FUNCTIONAL MATURATION DURING RENAL ORGANOGENESIS

We have only fragmentary knowledge of the developmental aspects of differentiation and the biochemical mechanisms that control and regulate the cellular events occurring during mammalian organogenesis. Some information on man is available, but considerably more on other mammals. The need for research in developmental biology directed toward defining more specifically the subcellular events underlying inductive membrane functions deserves mention here if only because biochemists are now showing a lively interest in reexamining the central importance of cell organization and the function of various membranes with the benefit of new techniques and models.[74] Considerable biochemical research is currently being pursued that is concerned with membrane function studies at the cellular and subcellular levels to define the nature of the integrated transport activity of specialized organized membrane systems. Studies of this kind have already yielded biochemical and biophysical data that have provided a new basis for understanding the well-recognized precision of biologic engineering in relating the specificity of structure and function at the cellular and subcellular levels in man and mammals.

The technique of isolating brush borders of hamster small intestine developed by Crane has been utilized by him and others to provide a much broader basis for understanding integrated activity of organized membrane systems with special reference to the brush border.[75] It is now apparent that the brush border is a structurally integrated, subcellular organelle, less complex perhaps but clearly of the same genre as mitochondria. This type of lining on a luminal surface epithelium provides a kinetic advantage for absorption, and major brush-border active-transport systems in the intestine are geared to the cellular sodium-ion transport mechanisms by a cooperative interaction between Na^+ and absorbed molecules such as amino acids and glucose. Comparable data are not presently available on brush-border activity in renal epithelium, but some of the knowledge gained by the study of intestinal brush border would presumably be applicable to the proximal renal tubule since sodium transport systems appear to be similar in both.

This aspect might be of great interest if methods were available to study brush-border activity of proximal renal tubules, especially with reference to the ontogenetic and developmental stages of kidney maturation in man and mammals. The studies cited earlier have demonstrated that the process of renal organogenesis is initiated by chemical reactions between cellular aggregates of two tissues when they possess the necessary specific and unique inductive capacity. These two "tissues" are developing in close proximity and are presumably separated by cell membranes necessary to mediate the chemically specific cellular and subcellular alterations that result in visible nephron induction. These primitive cellular organelles apparently have membranes possessing chemically specific functions that serve to direct subsequent differentiation of the complete nephron including the glomerulus and its unique vascular supply. It would appear that studies directed at defining the nature and the role of "inducers" in cellular differentiation can be pursued in the developing kidney with great likelihood of fruitful gain.

Some brief mention of the fragmentary knowledge available concerning the biochemical changes occurring at the cellular level in early organogenesis of the nephrons seems appropriate here. The mouse[25] has been more thoroughly studied than man. The mesonephros develops tubules that resemble those of the metanephros, but does not develop clearly defined brush borders or the high activity of cytoplasmic alkaline phosphatase at the luminal border that is characteristic of the secretory tubule of the metanephric kidney in the mouse or man. Such evidences of secretory activity do develop in mammals where the mesonephros has an excretory function (such as the pig, rabbit, or sheep). While the tubules of the mesonephros loop and curve, they do not branch. No open lumen was ever observed at the junction of the Wolffian duct with the cloaca. These findings are all in keeping with the view that the mesonephros is not functional as an excretory organ in the mouse.

The study of the ultrastructure of nephrons during human development and in the neonatal period by the use of electron microscopy has not been actively pursued. Vernier and Smith[76] noted that some of the proximal tubules in the human fetus resemble the adult structure. The brush border is less complex, the mitochondria are small, and numerous large round bodies which resemble lysosomes are present. The distal tubules are remarkable for the simplicity of the basilar membrane organization, but otherwise are very similar to the adult distal nephron.

Synthesis of ribonucleic acid (RNA) is known to be intimately associated with differentiation because of its important role in regulating cellular protein synthesis. Its localization in developing organs has been used as a "marker" of cell differentiation in developing organs. Vetter and Gibley[25] reported that in the developing mouse mesonephros the cytoplasm of the tubules showed the most marked basophilia (demonstrated histochemically to be RNA) during initial tubule formation. The basophilia became reduced when tubules reached maximum morphologic development. In the chick[77] and mouse metanephros the concentration and localization of RNA is heaviest in the secretory portions of the tubules. The absence of similar findings in the developing mesonephric tubule adds support to the view that the mesonephros does not acquire functional significance (as an excretory organ) in the mouse.

Alkaline phosphatase activity is known to play an important functional role in membrane and brush-border metabolic transport. Histochemical demonstration of its appearance at the luminal surface of epithelial cells involved in molecular transport has been interpreted as evidence of cell differentiation in developing organs. The early appearance and localization of these histochemical indications of cell differentiation in the mesonephros and the metanephros has been used to provide indirect evidence of a functional capability for membrane transport.[25,78] Many workers have studied the uptake of vital dyes in the developing avian and mammalian metanephros.[32,68,79,80] Wislocki found that the time of appearance of dye in the proximal renal tubular cells in the guinea pig fetus[81] and in the cat[82] could be correlated with the appearance of the brush border of the proximal tubular cells.

A correlation has also been found between dye uptake and anatomic evidence of development of proximal tubules undergoing maturation in the young rat using the vital dye trypan blue. Von Möllendorff[83] showed that this dye is stored by cells of the mature proximal convoluted tubule of the kidney during its excretion. In the rat, unlike man, new nephron production continues for 3 to 4 weeks after birth in the outermost layer of the cortex.

Baxter and Yoffey[84] studied the pattern of storage of this vital dye in the rat cortex during postnatal development. They found that no dye was stored in the peripheral neogenic zone of undifferentiated tissue, while the deeper nephrons did store dye. They correlated the ability of the renal tubules to store dye with tubular maturation and the acquisition of a brush border. These changes indicating functional and anatomic maturation of tubules were concomitant with maturation of the glomeruli, evident by thinning of the basement membrane and lobulation. They could identify by this means which of the peripheral cortical tubules are not fully developed or functional at birth. The pattern of protein and nucleic acid synthesis in fetal metanephric kidney late in gestation and in the newborn period in mice has been described by Priestley and Malt[85] and is considered in detail in Chapter 5.

CONCLUSIONS

Oliver's architectonic theory of renal development is a major advance and its foundation is biologically modern. It presumes that the developmental process of renal organogenesis occurs through critically phased steps of differentiation regulated at the cellular level and does not involve a series of trial-and-error events that are somehow self-adjusting. His development of a regulated sequential program describing renal development by means of quantitative data provides a growth blueprint identifying the most important developmental landmarks denoting the critical stages responsible for normal orderly embryonic growth of the metanephros into a mature kidney.

This new architectonic theory of renal development provides a basis for future studies aimed at unraveling the complex phenomenon causing polycystic and dysplastic aberrations in renal organogenesis. A new approach seems desirable since these malformations presently defy comprehensible classification in meaningful or etiologic terms. The complex events involved, together with a new concept of the "bioengineering" responsible for the maturation of the normal kidney, have been described in some detail with the hope of lessening our confusion about the factors that are of primary significance in producing malformations at the structural and/or functional level. It should be readily apparent that answers to the important questions raised when an explanation of structural malformations is attempted can be useful only to the extent that they deal with the complexity of organogenesis in modern terms. The tools used cannot involve one dimension when we are dealing with a multidimensional problem.

A classification of structural abnormalities based on morphologic criteria alone is arbitrary and will not reveal functional criteria or explain how the end result arose. All attempts to categorize polycystic disease on the basis of anatomic location (cortical or medullary) are doomed to failure in view of the complex final spatial arrangements of the various portions of the nephrons and collecting ducts and the devious pathways followed in the various stages of renal architectonic evolution. Even the tools of microdissection used by morphologists do not provide a solution to this problem, since the vital relations between structure and function cannot be defined simultaneously. It is to be hoped that new developments in biochemical techniques will allow a multifaceted attack to be launched, one that employs methods for defining functional characteristics (tissue markers, for example) that depend on cellular capacity for specific biochemical activities, such as H^+ or NH^+ secretion or transport of organic acids (amino acids and p-aminohippurate), as well as morphologic characteristics.

The demonstration by Burg and Orloff[86] that suspensions of isolated renal tubules can be utilized to study specific functional attributes is a stimulating development. They showed that these isolated renal tubules from rabbit renal cortex concentrated p-aminohippurate (PAH), consumed oxygen, and maintained normal concentration gradients for sodium and potassium for periods of several hours. This preparation has subsequently been used to study PAH uptake,[87] PAH efflux,[88] galactose uptake,[89] and amino acid uptake.[90]

As our knowledge of the unique functional characteristics of the various portions of the nephrons and collecting ducts increases, the use of techniques of this kind with microdissection may provide new and essential information needed for the taxonomy required to decipher the presently untranslatable renal parenchymal malformations. The use of the developing mammalian kidney as an experimental model for the study of the basic processes underlying normal organ differentiation will also be useful if we are to define the causes of malformation, since this information cannot readily be obtained in man.

Plates 1.1 through 1.9 reproduced by permission of Jean Oliver and Harper and Row from Dr. Oliver's monograph, *Nephrons and Kidneys: A Quantitative Study of Developmental and Evolutionary Mammalian Renal Architectonics* (New York: Hoeber Medical Division, Harper and Row, 1968).

PLATES

PLATE 1.1.   Earliest evidence of vesicle induction and the rudimentary nephron.
(A) A divided collecting tubule (*Col.T.*) ends in two ampullae (*Amp.*). At the
lower left, the earliest evidence of vesicle formation is seen in the proliferation of
a closely attached, disc-like mass of deeply stained nephrogenic mesenchyme; no
central cavity is visible. Attached below to the ampulla is the connecting tubule
(*C.T.*) of a previously induced nephron. Above and to the right is an ampulla with
a small but fully developed spherical vesicle in which a central cavity can be dimly
seen through its multicellular wall. (Specimen 1099, 6¼ months; magnification ca.
380.) (B) Above and to the left of the bilobed ampulla is a more mature vesicle
with a multicellular wall and large concentric central cavity. Transaction by the
dissecting needle has separated it slightly from the ampulla to reveal the firmness
of its attachment. (Same specimen and magnification as Plate 1.1A.) (C) The
deepened grooves and the proliferation of the tubule between them delineate
Stoerk's complex and the glomerular anlage (*arrow*). The continuous lumen of
the vesicle-nephron is barely apparent in the central portion of Stoerk's complex but
it is evident in the connecting tubule (*C.T.*) and within the glomerular anlage,
where it will eventually take the form of Bowman's space. (Specimen 1131,
6 months; magnification ca. 380.)

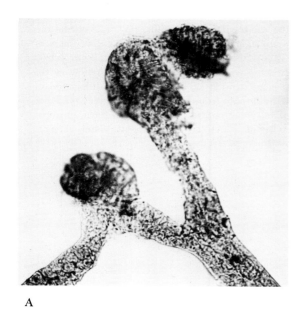

A

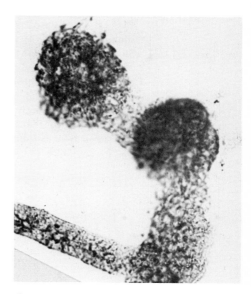

B

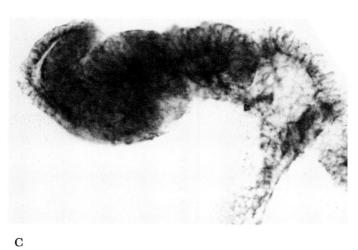

C

PLATE 1.2. Vascularization of the rudimentary glomerulus. (A) The needle has slightly separated the glomerular cup (*GL*) from the bilobed (*a* and *b*) mass of Stoerk's complex (*St.Comp.*) revealing the anlage of the proximal convolution (*P.C.*) and the vascularized mesenchyme which has grown into the hollow of the cup. (Specimen 1099, 6¼ months; magnification ca. 380.) (B) The dislocation of the two coils (*a* and *b*) of Stoerk's complex from the glomerular cup (*GL*) has occurred spontaneously, and the edges of the cup have extended to form an ovoid hemisphere into the still-open cavity of which a thick afferent vessel extends. (Specimen 1099, 6¼ months; magnification ca. 380.)

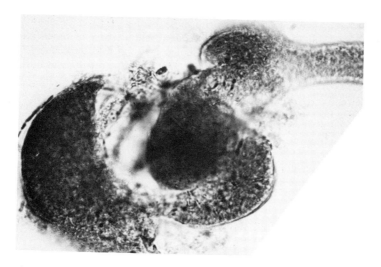

A

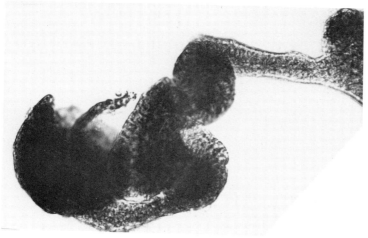

B

PLATE 1.3. Nephron luminal development and growth. (A) Considerable detail can be seen of the continuous lumen from the large central space of Stoerk's complex through the proximal convolution and its extension as thin dark line (2) of Bowman's space where the growth of the tuft (1) has compressed it against the epithelium of the external capsule (3). Extending into the anlage of the tuft a sharply outlined small vessel is apparent (*arrow*). (Specimen 1155, 7½ months; magnification ca. 390.) (B) A collecting tubule divides, ending in two terminal ampullae. The one to the left shows beginning budding division; in the one to the right division is imminent, as indicated by the notch at its apex. To each are attached two nephrons of differing ages. On the left they have the common attachment of an early arcade and on the right the connecting tubules are contiguous but still individual. Contrasting with the narrow collecting tubule with its regularly distributed cellular pattern of columnar epithelium are the proliferating masses of irregularly distributed cells which lie beneath (*left*) and surround (*right*) the attachments of the nephrons to the ampullae (*arrow*). The position of this exuberant growth is similar to that shown in Peter's hypothetical diagram, Fig. 1.8. (Specimen 1117, 3¾ months; magnification ca. 190.)

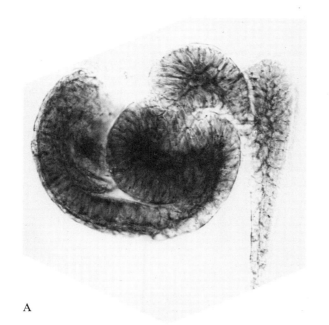

A

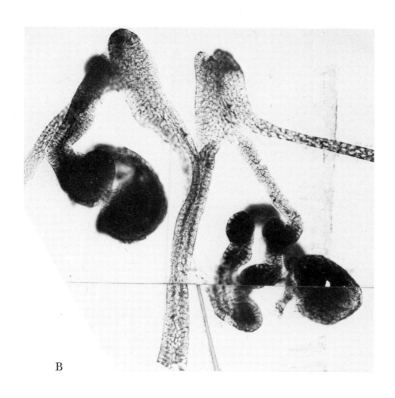

B

PLATE 1.4.   The arterial system of the kidney at 2¾ months. The dissection shows that by the end of the second month the general configuration of the arterial system of the adult organ has been established. From an arcuate artery (A) an interlobular branch (B) ascends toward the surface of the kidney, emitting lateral branches which end as the afferent arterioles of the glomeruli. At (C) an afferent passes from a branch of the arcuate artery to a glomerulus which lies in what would be described in the adult kidney as the juxtamedullary zone. To the right above (D) are the capillary ramifications of the intertubular network of the cortex in which the glomeruli lie and into which their efferents drain. (Specimen 1106, 2¾ months; magnification ca. 94.)

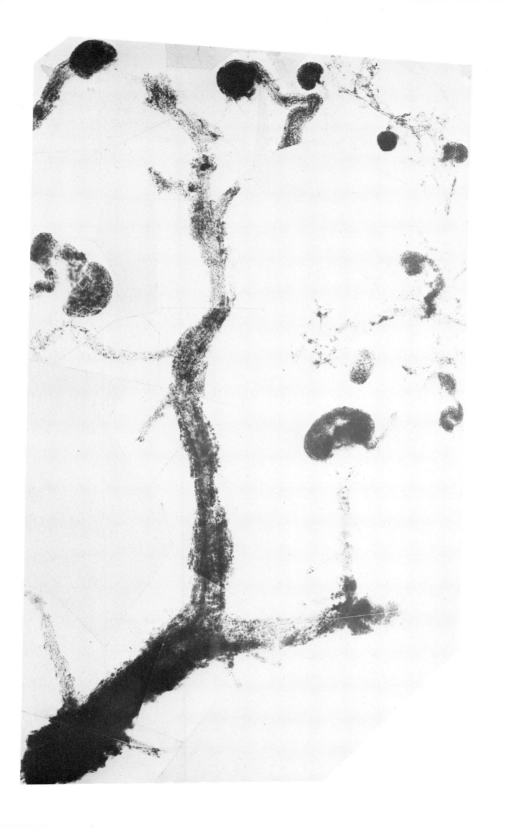

PLATE 1.5.   The collecting tree and nephrons at 2½ months. Two collecting trees arise from the calyx; four others have been removed. The general impression is of widely ramifying and dividing ducts, on the peripheral endings of which nephrons in varying stages of development have been induced. The pleomorphic configuration of the nephrons is the result of their unrestricted growth. In their recently induced form they have the same regular configurations as are seen in nephrons arising at later periods.

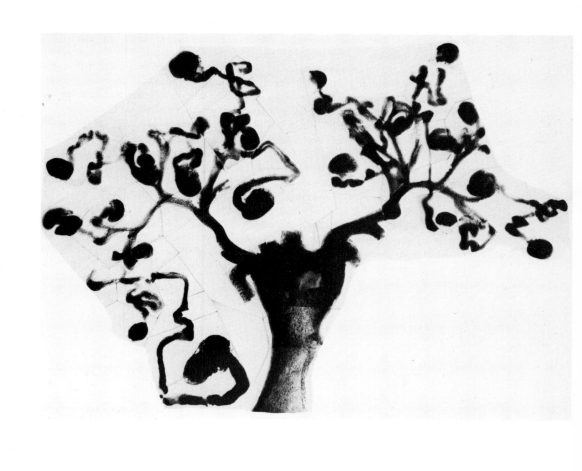

PLATE 1.6. The attachment of connecting tubule to the collecting duct. (A) A nephron with the configuration of Stoerk's complex is attached by its connecting tubule (*C.T.*) to a collecting tubule (*Col.T.*) which shows an incipient terminal bud. In its lowermost portion, the continuous lumen of the collecting tubule is seen to have arisen by an alignment of its epithelial cells, which are outlined by the dye remaining in the intercellular spaces after differentiation. The line of a definite luminal space becomes less certain as one ascends, and at (*a*) an indication of its division is apparent: one branch continues upward to the space of the protruding bud (*Amp.*), the other, inclining to the left, fades into the original random arrangement of the cells which compose the solid connecting tubule. At no focal plane in this region was there an indication of cellular alignment and a consequent lumen, the structure at this point being a solid cord of unoriented cells. Note that wherever alignment of the epithelial cells of the tubular wall is apparent— in the bud of the ampulla, the distal convolution, the tubule of Stoerk's complex, and the anlage of the proximal convolution—lumina have formed. (Specimen 1099, 6¼ months; magnification ca. 500.) (B) The regular alignment of the cells in the connecting tubule, which extends from the large central space of Stoerk's complex to the ampulla of the collecting duct, is visible as a darkly stained double line.

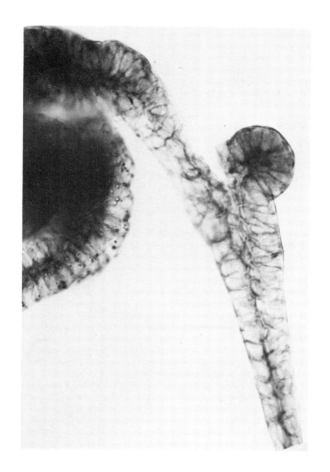

A

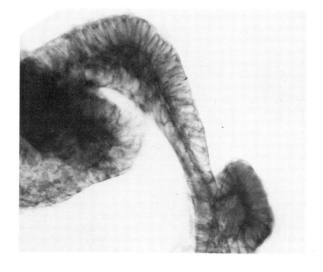

B

PLATE 1.7. A primitive calyx and provisional ducts from the kidney at 2⅛ months. The anterior wall of the calyx has been torn by the dissection at several places (x), revealing the central cavity. From this common space three large oval openings (a, b, and c) lead into the wide primitive ducts (A, B, and C). The two adjacent ducts on the right (B, C) arise from a common depression ($b + c$) and are separated by a fold of epithelium (d) which fades out on the posterior wall of the cavity of the calyx; the remnant of a similar fold is seen (e) below the opening (a) which leads to duct A on the left. The three primitive ducts are disproportionately wide, one-half the diameter of the calyx: that on the left (A) has divided (1) and then divided again (2); an oval recently induced vesicle (V) with its large central cavity is seen above, while below is an attached nephron of primitive configuration, though its various segments can be distinguished. Duct B ends in a complex which is to form a carrefour; there are two divisions (circled 1 and 2) and two incipient buds ($arrows$) which by extension will form branches and thus a central space with four radiating tubules. On the left is a nephron still tightly coiled in its early configuration; to the right is an induced vesicle with its large central cavity. Duct C ends in a bulbous projecting ampulla to which is attached a nephron; note that at this early stage of the development of the kidney the communication between the lumen of the duct and the connecting tubule of the nephron has already been established. At the arrow there is a mass of lightly stained proliferating cells which indicates the position of an incipient bud. Above is an attached nephron which has been spread apart by dissection; the typical early lengthening of its connecting tubule is apparent. The nephrons in this specimen are attached to ducts which are separated by only two divisions from the calyx; in the 2½-month specimen (Plate 1.5), where six divisions have occurred, the ducts are bare of nephrons up to their terminal divisions.

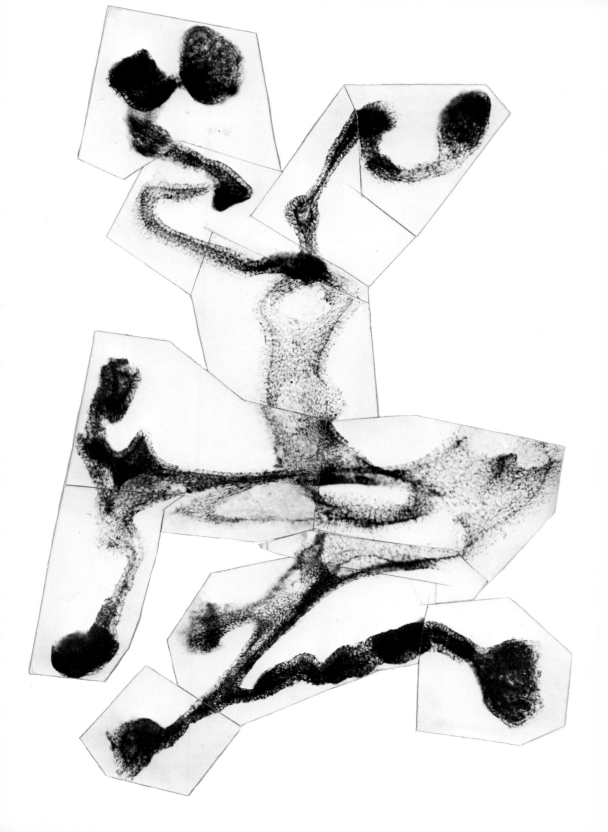

PLATE 1.8. Collecting tree at 3¾ months. Specimen 1117, 3¾ months. The widely divergent pattern of ductal growth is still evident with a marked pleomorphic configuration in the older nephrons. The ducts have divided seven and eight times to give rise to the origins of the XIIIth and XIVth generations.

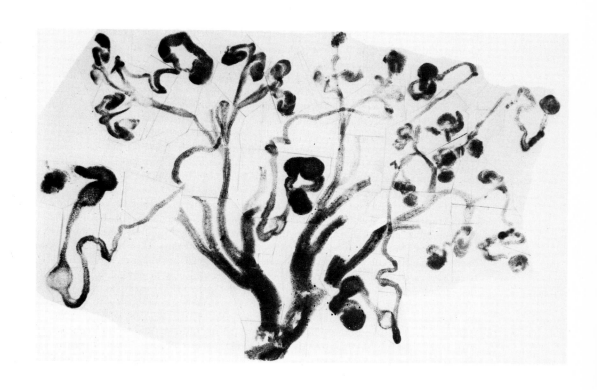

PLATE 1.9 The collecting tree at 5 months. Specimen 1118. This kidney 1¼ months older than that in Plate 1.8, weighed three times more and was approximately two-and-a-half times longer from the origin of the collecting tree at the papillary duct to the surface of the kidney. Accompanying this increase in size is a considerable degree of maturity in the general pattern of the tree. The ducts have divided nine times in all instances except four (*E* to *H*, 8 divisions) thus forming the final XVth generation of the ductal system; that is, its *closed divided portion* has thus been established. The divisions are now all bifid, but evidence of the correction of an earlier irregularity (trifid division) is noted on the right (*L*), where after the dichotomous division *4* there follows a very short generation (Xth) paired with a long branch. All the nephrons have been transported by Peter's intercalated zone of localized interstitial growth (Plate 1.3B) to the periphery and a suggestion of cortex and medulla is apparent. The nephrons appear in all their configurations from vesicles to those with well-developed loops of Henle; the former occur only at the surface on the terminal budding ampullae, never laterally to the ducts. Note that every nephron is attached to an ampulla either directly by its connecting tubule or by an arcade; none has lagged behind attached laterally to an earlier generation of a duct. Though a cortex can now be distinguished from the medulla, the demarcation is not sharply defined. The "cortex" at this point of development is not the equivalent of, or even structurally analogous to, that of the definitive adult kidney, as it includes only the *closed divided portion* of the collecting system. It contains only about one-third the ultimate number of nephrons. The remainder are to form on the *open direct portion* of the collecting system. The cortical region as it exists at this time, therefore, will form only the juxtamedullary zone of the definitive cortex.

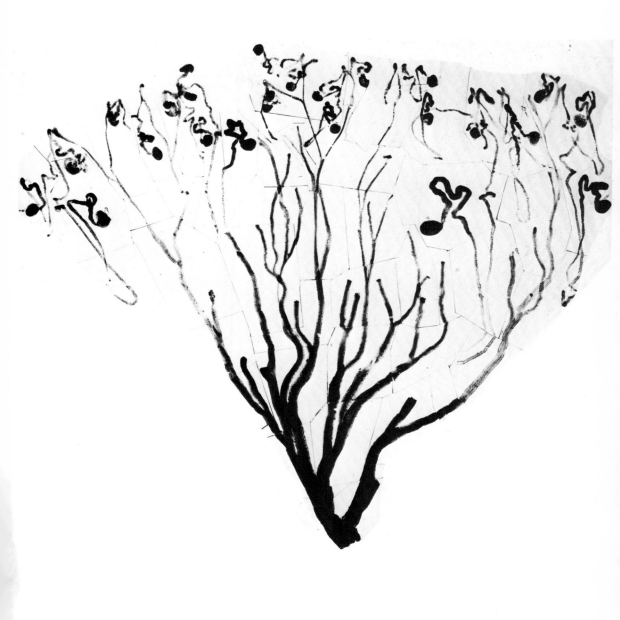

Chapter 2. Development of Renal Function in Utero

Needham[1] credits Leonardo da Vinci with being the first to observe that the human fetus forms urine in utero. The first reports on the composition of human urine formed in utero were those of Sabrazès and Fauquet[2] and Makepeace and his associates.[3] These authors were concerned with the origin of amniotic fluid and reported that fetal urine was hypotonic to plasma and similar in osmolar concentration to amniotic fluid. Considerations of this subject from the point of view of modern concepts of renal function have been presented by Alexander and Nixon[4] and more recently by Vernier and Smith.[5]

RENAL FUNCTION IN EARLY EMBRYOLOGIC LIFE

The exact time of onset of renal function during fetal life in man is conjectural. The metanephric kidney begins to differentiate at about the fifth week. The time of onset of secretory activity can be assumed a priori to occur after differentiation of the first functional nephrons. Gersh,[6] on the basis of evidence of morphologic differentiation that he correlated in other mammalian embryos (pig and cat) with direct evidence of tubular function, concluded that it begins in the human at about the ninth week of fetal life.

Oliver (see Plate 1.7) has provided clear anatomic evidence that function can be present at this early date. He found well-differentiated nephrons communicating with open collecting ducts in the youngest fetal kidney specimen (9 weeks) he examined. Hutchinson and his co-workers[7] proved that the fetal kidneys were functioning at 12 weeks of gestation by noting the sharp rise in isotope content in fetal urine after maternal administration prior to vaginal hysterectomy. Cameron and Chambers[8] provided the first direct evidence of human embryonic tubular functional capability by their demonstration in vitro that metanephric proximal tubules in fetal tissue culture explants have the ability to carry out active transport, as shown by their active uptake of phenol red and orange G dyes from the media and their ability to maintain a lower pH in tubular fluid than in the medium. The tissue they used was obtained from the kidney of a 14-week human fetus.

The pronephric tubules never become functional in mammalian embryos.[9] The mesonephric kidney functions in all mammals during early development, but Bremer[10] has shown that the size it attains and the time during fetal life when it has functional significance vary greatly in different species. In some species (for instance, man and the rat) the mesonephros appears early, develops a small number of functioning tubules attached to vascularized glomeruli, and then degenerates as the metanephric kidney forms. In others (including the sheep, pig, and rabbit) it becomes large enough to be a prominent abdominal organ in early fetal life with many tubules attached to glomeruli. Bremer's studies of the interrelations between the mesonephros, allantois, and placenta in different species showed that in general the size and functional importance of the mesonephros is directly related to that of the allantois. The mesonephros and allantois are largest in those forms which have a simple appositional type of placenta, which is presumably less effective for rapid removal of excretory products from the embryo into the maternal circulation. In primates, where the placenta is of the highly permeable hemochorial variety, the mesonephros is short-lived and the allantois is a mere diverticulum of the hindgut.

We can form some idea of the functional ability of the mesonephros from data on the composition of urine from the mesonephros of fetal pigs and sheep. The mesonephric urine represents a glucose- and protein-free fluid similar to an ultrafiltrate of fetal serum,[11,12] since the urea and solute concentration is similar to fetal plasma. Davies,[13] after studies of the mesonephros and metanephros in a number of anamniotes and avian, reptilian, and mammalian forms, commented that the metanephric kidney with its capacity to dilute or concentrate urine probably emerged in ontogenesis as the organism faced increasing environmental needs to conserve water. The metanephros replaced the mesonephros as the "final" kidney in land mammals because it provided an adaptation with survival value by supplying the necessary functional ability to adapt to the water-conserving requirements of terrestrial life where water is relatively scarce.

We do know something about the composition of mammalian fetal urine after the metanephros has become functional. Examination of the composition of fetal bladder urine in the lamb,[14,15] rabbit and pig,[16] and man[17] indicates that the fetal metanephric kidney elaborates what we consider to be true urine early in gestation in the sense that it differs characteristically in composition from a simple protein-free ultrafiltrate of plasma. It is slightly acidic, essentially free of glucose and protein, and is hypotonic to plasma with respect to the concentration of solute and sodium and chloride. It has a higher concentration of urea and creatinine than fetal plasma (urine-to-plasma ratio >1.0).

COMPOSITION OF HUMAN FETAL URINE

Reports analyzing the constituents of urine in early human fetal life are difficult to find. McCance and Widdowson[17] found that urine obtained from nonviable fetuses of 10 to 22 weeks of fetal age all had osmolar concentrations hypotonic to fetal plasma (115 to 217 mOsm/l), as is known to be the case in urine formed in utero just before normal birth. Vernier and Birch-Andersen,[18] in examining urine specimens (obtained from eleven human fetuses 12 to 19 weeks of fetal age) for protein, found all but two protein-free—and those two had only a trace of protein. There was no mention of other constituents.

The composition of urine formed in utero just before birth at term was determined by McCance and Widdowson[17] in twelve infants (three of whom were delivered by Caesarian section) and fetal serum and maternal serum were also examined. The mean values for the major constituents of urine are shown in Table 2.1.

It is apparent that urine passed by the infants immediately after birth, and presumably formed in utero, differed from that passed during the first 24 hours after birth and presumably formed ex utero. There were also marked differences apparent between the composition of infants' urine formed in utero and simultaneously formed maternal urine. This is of interest in view of the fact that maternal and fetal serum obtained simultaneously were essentially identical with respect to the concentration

TABLE 2.1   Composition of serum and urine in mother and infant at birth (from R. A. McCance and E. M. Widdowson[17])

| | Serum | | Urine | | |
| | | | | Infant | |
Component[a]	Mother	Infant cord	Mother	In utero	After birth
Osmolar concentration (mOsm/l)	303	300	698	137	317
Urea (mg%)	9.5	9.5	543	47.6	272
Creatinine (mg%)	0.9	1.1	139	5	64
Phosphate (mg%)	4.0	5.8	—	0	1.8
Sodium (mEq/l)	139	139	146	44	35.8
Chloride (mEq/l)	106	105	154	41.4	46.1
Potassium (mEq/l)	5.0	6.8	98	4.7	35

[a] All values represent average of twelve samples in each group.

of all of the measured constituents. Fetal urine formed in utero was hypotonic, while maternal urine formed simultaneously was hypertonic.

There is clear evidence that a relative water diuresis was present in the infant in utero. The fetal kidney was excreting hypotonic urine with a low urea and creatinine urine-to-plasma (U/P) ratio (about 5) indicating that about 20 percent of filtered water was being excreted. In contrast, maternal urea and creatinine U/P ratios were high (57 and 155 respectively), indicating that 1 percent or less of the filtered water was being excreted and reflecting a condition of antidiuresis with elaboration of hypertonic urine.

The babies' urine formed in utero had lower concentrations of sodium, potassium, and chloride than the maternal urine. Inorganic phosphate was essentially absent from fetal urine in spite of the fact that the fetal serum has a higher concentration of inorganic phosphate than the maternal serum. The fraction of total urinary osmolar concentration accounted for by urea in fetal urine formed in utero was quite low (28 percent) compared to that found in maternal urine (77 percent) or the infant's urine passed after birth (85 percent). In the absence of measurements of the rate of urine flow, no meaningful comments can be made about the rate of excretion of electrolytes. Filtered inorganic phosphate is, however, clearly being essentially completely resorbed by the fetal kidney.

The first urine formed ex utero was slightly hypertonic to plasma. The increase in the U/P ratio for urea and creatinine observed after birth (urea U/P = 28, creatinine U/P = 58) indicates that an increase in the rate of tubular water resorption occurred, resulting in a decrease in the fraction of filtered water excreted immediately after birth to 2 percent as compared to the higher fraction (20 percent) excreted prior to birth in utero. The increases in urine concentration of urea, potassium, and phosphate without comparable changes in sodium and chloride after birth were attributed by McCance and Widdowson[17] to the protein catabolic effects of the stress response these infants experienced with delivery. Of special interest from the standpoint of renal function, however, is evidence indicating that the kidney at term has the capacity to exhibit a functionally significant degree of antidiuresis (elaboration of a hypertonic urine) and appears to be responding to the fetal intrauterine environment prior to birth by a water diuresis elaborating a hypotonic urine. More will be said about this later.

QUANTITATIVE MEASUREMENTS OF RENAL FUNCTION DURING FETAL LIFE

There are obvious technical limitations to the use that can be made of data derived from random samples of bladder urine and amniotic fluid to define the functional ability of the fetal kidney. The data on electrolyte composition of bladder urine can be misleading if urine has been retained in the bladder for long periods of time ("stale urine") because movement of water and electrolytes across the bladder wall can occur in response to electrolyte concentration gradients existing between urine and plasma.[19]

Techniques have recently been developed[15,20] which greatly extend the scope of investigations of fetal renal function by permitting the measurement of rates of urine flow and systematic study of fetal renal function. The preparation involves removing the fetus from the uterus but maintaining its placental circulation intact and avoiding its exposure to air. This preparation permits independent sampling of maternal and fetal blood during experimental observations (see Fig. 2.1). The preparation is spoken of as the exteriorized fetus and has been elegantly employed by Alexander and Nixon (using lambs) to provide most of the quantitative information presently available on renal function prior to birth.[4,21,22]

In any situation in which the placental circulation is intact (as in

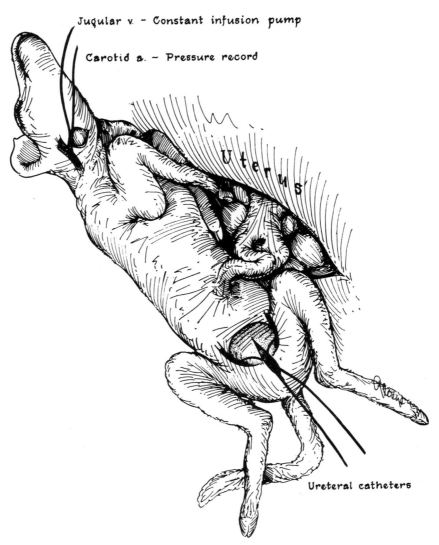

Jugular v. - Constant infusion pump

Carotid a. - Pressure record

Uterus

Ureteral catheters

FIGURE 2.1   Intact fetal-maternal preparation for studies of fetal renal function. The exteriorized but nonbreathing lamb fetus is shown lying adjacent to the ewe uterus with the umbilical circulation intact. Catheters have been placed in both ureters and in the external jugular vein for infusion and the internal carotid artery for blood sampling. (From F. G. Smith, Jr. et al.[24])

the exteriorized fetus) the concentration of water and electrolytes in fetal blood will be determined principally by placental transfer rates responding to conditions existing in the maternal environment. It is essential, therefore, to consider both the maternal and fetal environments in any attempt to interpret mechanisms regulating fetal renal function in utero. While recognizing that one cannot extrapolate findings in sheep and pigs directly to man, it nonetheless seems probable that the patterns of development of metanephric function in mammals would be qualitatively similar during intrauterine life. The data in these mammals are of great interest because we have no comparable data in man.

Changes in Urine Flow, C_{IN}, and C_{PAH} during Fetal Growth

The exteriorized sheep fetus has been used to provide the only quantitative data available on rate of urine formation and values for clearance of inulin (C_{IN}) and clearance of p-aminohippurate (C_{PAH}) in utero. The mesonephros has degenerated in fetal sheep by 60 days, so that urine passed thereafter is of metanephric origin.[23] Alexander and her associates[15] reported that fetal urine flow increased steadily from 0.14 ml/min at 61 days gestation to a high of 0.64 ml/min at 117 days, after which it declined to 0.14 ml/min just before term (145 days). When they related urine flow to body weight, it decreased with increasing gestational age; a similar finding has been observed in comparable studies in the guinea pig by Boylan, Colbourn, and McCance.[20]

The gradual increase in kidney weight that occurs with increasing gestational age would be expected to be associated with a parallel increase in glomerular filtration rate (GFR) and renal plasma flow (RPF) and in tubular transport capacity. Only data on the first two aspects of renal function during fetal growth in lambs are available. The values found by Alexander and Nixon[21] for C_{IN} and C_{PAH} in sheep (see Table 2.2) are expressed both as actual values and as ml/min/kg of body weight. This practice makes evaluation of changes in renal function as reflected in change of values for these plasma clearances difficult to compare with those in man, where plasma clearances have been related to a standard unit of body surface area (1.73 m² S.A.). An increase in the C_{IN} value per unit of body weight does, however, indicate that renal function is increasing at a faster rate than body weight as a whole, a change compatible with the expected development of progressively increasing renal functional ability per unit of body mass as gestation advances.

The values for C_{IN} and C_{PAH} shown in Table 2.2 both increased with

TABLE 2.2   Renal clearances in fetal, neonatal, and adult sheep (from D. P. Alexander and D. A. Nixon[21])

Subjects	Age	Number of cases	C_{IN}		C_{PAH}		FF
			ml/min	ml/min/kg	ml/min	ml/min/kg	C_{IN}/C_{PAH}
Fetuses	89–119 days	4	0.4(0.2–0.8)	0.5(0.4–0.8)	0.5(0.2–0.9)	0.6(0.5–0.8)	0.83
	121–140 days	5	1.7(0.8–2.2)	0.6(0.4–0.8)	2.3(1.2–2.8)	0.9(0.5–1.3)	0.67
	Full term	1	4.3	0.9	6.4	1.3	0.69
Lambs	1 day	1	9.0	4.5	12.5	6.3	0.71
	4 days	1	14.0	3.5	18.7	4.7	0.74
	13 days	1	11.4	3.5	22.1	6.7	0.52
Adults		3	91.4(55.3–138)	2.8(1.9–3.2)	417(300–645)	12.7(10–19.6)	0.22

Figures in parentheses indicate range of values obtained.
C_{IN} = clearance of inulin; C_{PAH} = clearance of p-aminohippurate.
FF = filtration fraction.

advancing gestational age whether expressed as actual rate or per kilogram of body weight. The values in ml/min/kg weight for C_{IN} at term were about one-third those of the adult animal on a comparable basis. The actual value doubled and the rate/min/kg weight quadrupled for both C_{IN} and C_{PAH} immediately following birth and separation from the placenta.

The value of C_{PAH} is surprisingly low when compared to that of C_{IN}, being only slightly greater than C_{IN} and thus resulting in a very high value of filtration fraction (C_{IN}/C_{PAH} = 0.63 to 0.89). It seems unlikely that this represents a valid estimate of either the true renal blood flow or fraction of plasma water filtered at the glomerulus. Little is known in any case about the dynamic interplay of glomerular filtration pressure, plasma protein oncotic pressure, and intrarenal pressure in the fetal kidney. The significance of the high value for the filtration fraction is thus obscure.

An estimate of the renal handling by the fetal kidney of creatinine has been provided by the finding of Alexander and Nixon[22] that the mean value for inulin/creatinine clearance ratios was similar in fetal lambs of 80 to 142 days (mean C_{IN}/C_{CR} = 1.45) to that found in mature nonpregnant ewes (mean C_{IN}/C_{CR} = 1.44). It would appear that some of the filtered creatinine is resorbed in the fetal nephron as is the case in the mature ewe. The fact that the placental circulation is intact in these studies of exteriorized fetal lambs introduces the possibility of error in the calculation of true fetal C_{IN} and C_{PAH}, because PAH and inulin could pass into the maternal circulation to be removed by the maternal kidney. Until we know what true renal blood flow (RBF) is, we cannot know what the true filtration fraction is in this situation.

The persistence of high values for the filtration fraction after birth is equally difficult to interpret. The usefulness of C_{PAH} as an estimate of renal blood flow will not be known until the renal PAH excretion of the fetal and young lamb kidney has been measured. The data are of some interest nonetheless because they provide the only available estimates of the magnitude of GFR and RBF during fetal growth. Smith and his associates,[24] using a technique comparable to that of Alexander and Nixon,[4] have found similar values for C_{IN} in fetal sheep. It is of interest that the filtration fraction remains high, falling only to 0.52 in newborn sheep up to 13 days of postnatal age, even though the actual values for both C_{IN} and C_{PAH} rise sharply immediately after birth (see Table 2.2). This can be interpreted as evidence that the renal handling of PAH by the fetal kidney changes slowly following separation of the placenta for at least the first few days after birth.

The explanation for the low values of C_{PAH} relative to C_{IN} with resulting high values of the filtration fraction is presently speculative. While methodologic errors inherent in the preparation used may play a significant role, one additional factor would presumably be that the tubular transport capacity for PAH is not so fully developed in the fetal proximal tubules as in the mature kidney. Direct measurement of renal tubular transport activity of renal cortical slices for PAH in fetal rabbits[25] and in puppies[26] has demonstrated that the tubular transport system seems to be underdeveloped in both, since the rate of accumulation of PAH/mg of tissue is less than that found with equivalent tissue from adult kidneys of the same species.

The values in the first week or two of neonatal life were interestingly even lower than those found with the fetal kidney. The explanation for this reduced uptake (that is, limited enzyme concentration or low activity) is not evident, but these findings suggest that cellular immaturity (incomplete differentiation) may be a major factor accounting for the reduced PAH transport capacity found in the fetal renal proximal tubular tissue. A second factor involves the possibility that distribution of intrarenal blood flow differs in the immature kidney from that in the mature kidney. It seems likely that in the fetal kidney a smaller proportion of renal blood flow is directed to the outer cortex—and the proximal tubules of those nephrons—and a greater proportion to the deeper nephrons and the juxtamedullary glomeruli which are more mature. If this is the case, the capacity for PAH secretion would be decreased since more blood would bypass the proximal tubules by flowing through the vasa recta and lowering the PAH extraction ratio (see Chapter 3).

The contribution of these two factors (immature tubular transport mechanisms and intrarenal circulatory bypass around proximal tubules) could explain the low values for C_{PAH}. An additional possibility would be that nutrient blood flow (perfusion of nonsecretory tissue) is proportionally greater in the immature lamb kidney than in the mature organ. The abrupt increase noted[21] in value for C_{IN} and C_{PAH} after birth of the lamb is of great interest nonetheless. It suggests that there is a marked increase in RBF and GFR immediately after birth.

Renal Blood Flow in the Perinatal Period

Direct measurements of fetal renal blood flow have demonstrated that total renal blood flow increases promptly and significantly after the fetus is separated from the placenta. Assali, Bekey, and Morrison[27] employed electromagnetic flow meters to record the magnitude of renal blood flow directly in terms of the fractional cardiac output delivered to various organs including the kidney in the exteriorized fetal lamb before and after lung expansion and cord clamping. They found proportional fetal renal blood flow relative to total flow to be low before placental separation, but immediately thereafter a redistribution of cardiac output occurred and renal blood flow increased.

Rudolph and Heymann[28] measured fetal circulation in utero by the technique of Meschia and his colleagues,[29] which does not involve exteriorizing the fetus during study, and also found low values in utero for renal blood flow (1.5 ml/gm/min, range 0.6 to 2.8) and an increase in the proportion of cardiac output delivered to the kidney after birth. The fetal kidneys thus appear to receive a considerably smaller fraction of the fetal cardiac output than is the case in extrauterine life. This situation appears to be unique to the fetal environment and prevails in certain other organs and regions as well. The placenta and fetal membranes receive the major portion of the fetal cardiac output (57 percent). A small proportion flows through the lungs (10 percent), to the head and foreparts (15 percent), and to the hindparts (18 percent).

Fetal umbilical arterial blood pressure has been shown to rise progressively in sheep[14] and in man[30] with increasing gestational age. The potential glomerular perfusion pressure could thus progressively increase during gestation even though renal afferent arteriolar resistance was maintained at a high level, limiting absolute GFR and RBF. One can conclude that the fetal renal vascular resistance must be maintained at high level, and a state of "relative" renal ischemia may be postulated to exist in utero in the fetal kidney.

Tubular Resorption of Salt and Water

The nephrons demonstrate increasingly efficient tubular resorption of electrolytes with increasing fetal age. The fractional rates of sodium and chloride resorption of the filtered load parallel each other from the earliest period of fetal life studied and increase continuously as gestation advances. The values for each rise from roughly 60 percent resorption of the filtered load at the earliest period of study (61 days) to 90 percent or greater resorption of filtered load at term.[12,14] Potassium excretion remains low and fairly constant (less than 20 percent of filtered load) throughout gestation. The resorption of filtered water parallels that of salt but is less complete.

TABLE 2.3   Average values for bladder urine in three fetal age ranges in sheep
(from D. P. Alexander and D. A. Nixon[4])

Fetal age (days)	Osmolar conc. (mOsm/l)	Urea	Creatinine	Phosphate	Na	Cl	K
			(mg/100 ml)			(mEq/l)	
81–93	239	102	3	9	81	67	4
104–117	207	123	6	2	71	47	4
130–142	116	287	27	3	26	21	8

The nephrons thus appear to develop the capacity to resorb an increasing fraction of glomerular filtrate as the fetal kidney develops and grows. This suggests that some degree of glomerulotubular balance develops as the nephrons mature. The creatinine and urea concentrations in fetal urine are always higher than those of fetal plasma and rise progressively as gestational age increases; this is shown in Table 2.3. The actual amount of urea and nitrogen found in fetal urine is low, however, in comparison to that typical of the mature subject. From the value of the creatinine U/P ratio (3 at 81 to 93 days and 5 to 20 at 130 to 142 days) the fractional resorption of filtered water can be estimated to approximate 33 percent at 81 to 93 days, rising to 80 to 95 percent late in gestation.[12,15]

The fact that there are consistent differences in fractional salt and water resorption is evident in the findings that the osmolar concentration of fetal urine is always lower than that of plasma throughout gestation and decreases as gestational age increases. The capacity of the nephrons to elaborate a urine hypotonic to fetal plasma is already evident at 81 to 93 days of fetal age, as indicated in the table. These findings constitute presumptive evidence that the loops of Henle in some nephrons are functioning early in fetal life. Active resorption of sodium in the ascending limb of Henle's loop without isoosmotic movement of water would be required to deliver dilute urine to the distal tubules and collecting ducts. If the medullary osmolar gradient were small and flow were high, there would be little subsequent concentration of urine in its passage through the distal nephron.

An alternative explanation is that the resorption of salt is greater than that of water in the distal nephrons and collecting ducts without benefit of selective sodium resorption by the loop of Henle and development of an active countercurrent mechanism to establish some degree of solute gradient in the medullary tissues. This would imply that limited membrane permeability to water exists in the distal portions of the nephrons but not in the ascending loops of Henle, which seems unlikely. There is no evidence to support the existence of such selectively reduced membrane permeability as a phenomenon of immaturity.

The data available suggest that the former theory is more likely. Gersh[6] provided qualitative evidence that tubular resorption of water occurs with maturation of nephrons, as evidenced by increased luminal dye concentration in the thin limb of the loop of Henle and continuing into the distal portions of the tubule in fetal kidneys of the cat and pig. He found that morphologic differentiation of the thick and thin limbs of the loop of Henle correlated closely with evidence of tubular function in all of the species he examined. On the basis of morphologic criteria he concluded that function could take place in the loop of Henle in the human metanephros by the thirteenth week of fetal life. The onset of function could be ascertained directly if we knew when a corticomedullary osmotic gradient develops in the fetal kidney.

Tubular unresponsiveness by the fetal nephron to antidiuretic hormone (ADH) has been postulated.[17] While it is true that the amount of ADH in the newborn is apparently minimal and thus presumably not available in the fetus,[31] maternal ADH could be present since it can apparently pass across the placenta. Vasopressin has been isolated from placental tissue along with a number of other polypeptide hormones of pituitary origin.[32] Still, there is no direct evidence available concerning the antidiuretic sensitivity of the fetal nephron to vasopressin. Alexander and Nixon[4] supported the idea that the fetal nephron was unresponsive to ADH and observed that the exteriorized sheep fetus near term could elaborate a hypertonic urine (610 mOsm/l), but intramuscular administration of vasopressin did not increase this value. They also noted, however, that urine in a 130-day-old fetus that became hypotonic during an induced diuresis became slightly hypertonic after intramuscular vasopressin; however, there was also a fall in glomerular filtration rate, so the result is difficult to interpret. The fact that the fetus is usually elaborating hypotonic urine is clearly not evidence that it does so because it lacks the capacity to form a hypertonic urine under any circumstances. The findings cited provide suggestive functional evidence that after structural maturation has occurred the fetal nephron is qualitatively similar to the mature nephron in possessing the ability to dilute and concentrate urine to some degree. The data available are, however, still too incomplete to allow a definite statement to be made on this complicated subject.

Tubular Resorption of Glucose

The capacity for tubular resorption of filtered glucose is present early in gestation. Urine is essentially free of glucose at the earliest ages examined in fetal pigs and sheep at normal plasma concentrations of glucose, while resorption of fructose is incomplete in both. Alexander and Nixon[33] showed that glucose resorption by the fetal nephrons is a result of active transport and is rate-limited. They demonstrated an increase in the rate of tubular absorption of glucose in fetal sheep when glucose was infused and did find a limiting threshold, although they were unable to define a reproducible tubular transport capacity for glucose ($Tm_{GLUCOSE}$). The rate of glucose absorption was markedly reduced by the administration of phlorhizin. The nephron may develop the capacity for active glucose transport at an early age, since histochemical evidence of alkaline phosphatase activity can be seen in the proximal tubule of the sheep metanephros as early as 43 days.

Renal Mechanisms for Urinary Acidification of the Fetal Kidney

The fetus lives in utero in a state of mild metabolic acidosis when compared to the adult.[34,35] The manner by which the fetal kidney handles hydrogen ions is not known. Renal acid excretion would not be vital in fetal acid-base homeostasis, which is ultimately regulated by the maternal lungs and kidneys. The fetal kidney has the ability to acidify urine since it is usually acidic (pH around 6).[36] This is about what might be expected if urine were to be bicarbonate-free and there were no great need for acid excretion. While fetal renal acid excretion into amniotic fluid does occur, attempts at defining relationships between changes in pH of the amniotic fluid and of the fetal blood have failed. The degree of metabolic acidosis in the fetus does not correlate with lowering of the pH of the amniotic fluid. Whether the fetal kidney plays any role in fetal acid-base homeostasis is unknown.

An attempt was made by Vaughn and his associates[37] to study the response of the fetal kidney to an acid load and to evaluate the relative contribution of the placenta and fetal kidneys to hydrogen ion excretion. They employed a technique involving marsupialization of the exteriorized fetus to the uterine wall.[38] The intravenous infusion of HCl at increasing rates was used to deliver the acid load. In the fetus this resulted in a prompt and consistent fall in fetal umbilical arterial blood pH and HCO_3, but pCO_2 was not consistently changed. Uterine venous blood became more acidic as well. The changes in umbilical venous blood were similar but less marked and pCO_2 actually rose. Fetal urine pH fell moderately in most instances, the lowest value being 5.45. The observed changes in urinary titratable acidity (TA) and NH_4 were, however, minimal or inconsistent, although instances were observed where there was a substantial increase in one or the other component.

These results support the view that the maternal kidneys and lungs play the major role in response of the fetus to acidosis, acting via the placenta. The same infusion in the newborn lamb produced a marked metabolic acidosis with a fall in arterial blood pH, HCO_3 and pCO_2; the changes observed in renal response were appropriate. The observed magnitude of the drop in urine pH and the increase in TA or NH_4 excretion correlated generally with the degree of acidosis induced. The lowest value noted for urine pH was 5.49. The overall response as judged by observed fall in urine pH was considerably reduced when compared to that observed with a similar acid load given to the adult ewe. While the authors attributed the absence of a consistent or significant renal response to renal immaturity, placental participation in this situation could partly explain the failure to observe a consistent metabolic acidosis or fall in pCO_2 in fetal lambs. These factors would tend to minimize the renal response in fetal lambs and the acid load would be largely removed via the placenta. The minimal fetal response is not surprising, since protection against rapid changes in fixed anion or hydrogen ion concentration in the fetus is provided for by the existence of a relatively slow rate of exchange of bicarbonate across the placenta as demonstrated by Blechner, Meschia, and Barron.[36]

By means of indwelling plastic catheters, without exteriorizing the fetus, these researchers measured the blood levels of pCO_2, pH, and HCO_3 in maternal and intrauterine fetal sheep in the "steady state" and after NH_4Cl infusion in the mother. They demonstrated that fetal pCO_2 is always higher than maternal arterial pCO_2 despite wide variations in pCO_2 in maternal blood. The bicarbonate level in fetal blood was relatively independent of acute changes in bicarbonate in maternal blood. There appeared to be slower diffusion of bicarbonate across the placenta; acute changes in pCO_2 may therefore result in changes in fetal pH in a direction opposite to that occurring in the maternal fluids.

More recently Smith and Schwartz[39] reported a similar study in which they succeeded in producing a consistent metabolic acidosis in the exteriorized fetal lamb (pH fell to a mean of 7.02, range 6.94 to 7.11) by infusion of hydrochloric acid, and they observed a clear-cut renal response to the acidosis. Following the induction of metabolic acidosis in the fetal lamb, urine pH fell to a mean value of pH 5.92 (range 5.5 to 6.25) from a mean control value of pH 7.26. Significant increase in urinary titratable acid and ammonium excretion occurred over control values in all subjects and phosphate excretion also rose significantly.

While this response to metabolic acidosis is quantitatively less than that observed in the adult ewe in a similar situation, it does demonstrate that the fetal lamb kidney has the capacity to increase hydrogen ion excretion significantly, and in a manner qualitatively similar to the adult animal, when presented with a significant degree of metabolic acidosis. The limitation in the renal response of the fetal lamb to acutely induced metabolic acidosis as judged by comparison with the fall in urine pH and rise in urinary titratable acid and ammonium excretion seen in the adult is usually ascribed to renal immaturity, but this is too general to provide much insight into the actual mechanisms involved.

One factor that could be involved in the limitation of the fetal kidney is the meager supply of urinary buffer available for acid excretion. It has already been mentioned that the fetal urine is essentially free of phosphate. The ability of the fetal nephron to achieve a marked hydrogen ion gradient between tubular epithelium and lumen may be limited, but no quantitative data bearing on this possibility are yet available. The fact that all of the fetal lambs in the studies of Smith and Schwartz acidified urine to some degree indicates that this limitation must also be qualitative. The factors regulating adaptation also deserve study, since the fetal environment does not place a stress on the fetal kidney comparable to that existing in extrauterine life with respect to removal of hydrogen ions.

Short-term studies of renal function in the exteriorized fetus have also been used to examine the functional state of one of the enzymatic steps involved in tubular bicarbonate resorption and hydrogen ion excretion required for renal acidification. The enzyme carbonic anhydrase is known to play an important role in tubular resorption of bicarbonate in the kidney. Smith, Tinglof, and Adams[40] demonstrated that the characteristic mature renal response to administration of a carbonic acid inhibitor can be observed in the fetal lamb. The parenteral administration of the carbonic acid inhibitor acetozolamide caused a prompt increase in urinary pH (from 7.0 to 7.8) and a tenfold increase in urinary bicarbonate content. Such a response indicates that one of the required enzymes involved in the normal mechanisms for renal tubular bicarbonate resorption is present and active before birth. This was probably to be expected since it has also been shown that the carbonic anhydrase activity of renal tissue of premature infants is similar to that of full-term infants and adults.[41]

Renal Tubular Responsiveness to Parathormone

The fetus and newborn have been shown to have a very low renal phosphate clearance and virtually no inorganic phosphate in the urine. The fetal plasma levels of inorganic phosphate are higher than those of maternal plasma.[14,24] This could be evidence that the fetal parathyroid gland is not active or that the renal tubule is not responsive to the phosphaturic effect of parathormone. The former would seem likely, since the levels of nonprotein-bound calcium are normal in fetal blood and in fact higher in fetal than in maternal blood in man and sheep.[42] Smith and his coworkers[24] have shown that the kidney of the fetal lamb does respond to exogenous parathormone with phosphaturia in a manner similar to that which I have demonstrated in the normal newborn.[43]

The fetal maternal phosphate gradient seems to be the result of an active process of placental uptake of phosphate, since Fuchs and Fuchs[44] found the rate of passage of phosphate from mother to fetus to be four times the rate of passage from fetus to mother. The fetus appears to be avidly retaining inorganic phosphate, possibly because of the high requirements for growth.[42] The fetal plasma phosphate concentration is apparently not subject to regulation by the rate of excretion of phosphate by the fetal kidney as is the case in the newborn after separation from the placenta. The newborn infant's well-recognized reduced ability for renal excretion of phosphate loads[43] can also be looked upon as a carry-over of its adaptation to the intrauterine environment.

WHAT IS THE PHYSIOLOGIC ROLE OF THE FETAL KIDNEY?

The fetal kidney has not been credited with any physiologic role in mammals except for the contribution of fetal urination to the volume and composition of the allantoic and amniotic fluids. Since the allantois is

relatively unimportant in primates, the role of fetal urination in the production of allantoic fluid will not be discussed even though it has been
the subject of investigation in sheep and pigs.[4,5,12] The significance of
fetal urination as a source of amniotic fluid is still minimized by some
investigators[17,45] but the data to be reviewed here, which have accumulated in the last ten years, on the composition of fetal urine and amniotic
fluid give strong support to the view that fetal urination in man is a
major source of amniotic fluid and influences its volume and composition
after the tenth to twelfth week of gestation.

The role of the fetal kidneys in the production of amniotic fluid has
been a subject of interest ever since Hippocrates postulated that the liquor
amnii represented fetal urine.[46] In sheep and pigs, fetal urine is passed
into the allantoic sac via the urachus until the patency of the urethra
is established.[10,13] It is then passed into the amniotic cavity as well and
continues to pass into the allantois until the urachus closes. In primates,
the situation is quite different. The amnion forms during the third week
of fetal life in man and the amniotic sac completely fills the chorionic
vessel at the end of the second month. This membrane is in direct contact
with the chorion but has no contact or connection with the allantois
even during the earliest stage of embryonic life.[47] The allantois is vestigial
in primates, as is the urachus.[10]

Since human fetal urine cannot gain access to the amniotic cavity
until after the onset of fetal renal function and after the patency of
the urethra is established (eighth to ninth week), it cannot contribute
to the initial formation of the amniotic fluid. It is presumably discharged
into the amniotic cavity sometime after the eighth to ninth week and
clearly must influence its composition during the rest of gestational life.

The composition of amniotic fluid is influenced by other more important routes whereby exchanges of fluid and electrolyte occur between
the fetal and maternal environments. The dynamics of fetomaternal fluid
and electrolyte exchange across the placental membranes thus require
comment in order that the contribution of fetal urine formation to the
composition of the amniotic fluid may be considered in proper perspective. The placental membranes are freely permeable to water, urea, and
electrolytes whose movement across the placenta is extremely rapid. As
a consequence, the osmolality and concentration of sodium, potassium,
bicarbonate, chloride, and urea of fetal and maternal blood are maintained essentially in equilibrium. This complex subject has been extensively reviewed by Assali and his associates[47] and only those factors in-

fluencing the function of the fetal kidney in utero will be considered here.

PLACENTAL PATHWAYS OF WATER AND SOLUTE EXCHANGE BETWEEN MOTHER AND FETUS

Bruns and his colleagues[48] demonstrated that the fetus participates in the fluid and solute transfers involved in correcting distortions in osmolar concentration of maternal fluids. They found that an acute increase in solute concentration induced in maternal plasma by mannitol infusion results in a prompt increase in fetal plasma solute concentration. There was a net movement of water out of the intracellular and extracellular fetal compartments into the mother as the distortion was corrected. In general, changes induced in the maternal volume of body water or plasma osmolar or sodium concentration were associated with prompt parallel alterations in fetal fluids.

Phillips and Sundaram[49] have shown that sodium depletion of pregnant ewes causes sodium depletion in the fetus. The concentration of sodium in fetal plasma and amniotic fluid was lower than that of controls and the volume of allantoic fluid was greater. This experiment suggests that the sodium-deficient fetus, like the sodium-deficient adult, responds to the deficiency by restricting urinary sodium losses and increasing urinary water excretion. Even though the response of the fetal kidney may be appropriate to the "internal" physiologic state existing in the fetus at a given time, its significance in effecting correction is negated because fetal urine is not eliminated from the fetal environment; instead it is retained in the amniotic cavity where it continues to influence the fetal and maternal environment.

In an effort to quantitate the kinetics of its water exchange, the fetus has been likened to a small fluid compartment existing within a three-compartment system that is maintained in fluid and electrolyte equilibrium with the maternal environment.[7] In the human at term the intrauterine water compartment accounts for 80 percent of the intrauterine contents by weight. The fetus represents 2,800 ml, the amniotic contents 700 ml, with the placenta accounting for 400 ml.[50] This compartment is small, however, in comparison to the total maternal pool, accounting for less than a tenth of the total body water of the mother at term. The fetoplacental unit can be likened to a multicompartmental system involving transfers between three fluid-filled compartments that exchange directly via transfer between: (1) fetal and maternal blood pools; (2) fetal fluids and the amniotic fluid; and (3) the amniotic fluid and the maternal pool, via direct transfer across placental membranes without the fetus acting as an intermedium.

Quantitative studies on the rates of water and electrolyte exchange have largely been carried out in primates because the opportunities for such studies in man are obviously limited. In the human the rate of water and electrolyte exchange via the placenta between the mother and fetus is very rapid. Hellman and his colleagues[51] investigated the exchange of water between mother and fetus, presumably via the placenta, and found that it increased progressively with increasing gestational age until term, when there was a sharp decline which they attributed to aging of the placenta. Hutchinson and his co-workers[7] found that the hourly exchange of water between the fetus and the mother via the placenta increases from about 100 ml/hr during the twelfth week to 3,000 to 4,000 ml/hr at term (see Fig. 2.2).

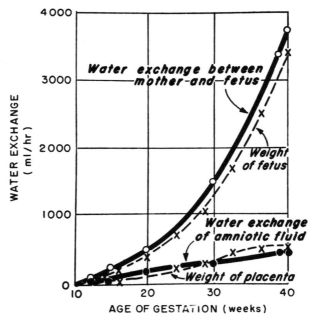

FIGURE 2.2   The relation of water exchange to age of gestation. The values are related to reported average values for fetal and placental weight in grams. (From D. L. Hutchinson et al.[7])

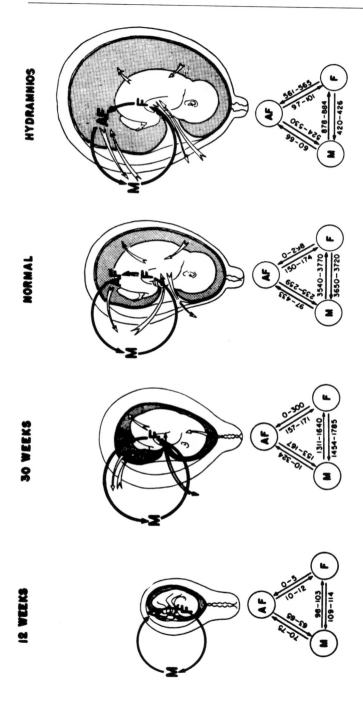

FIGURE 2.3 Schematic presentation of the water exchange between mother (M), fetus (F), and amniotic fluid (AF) in normal and pathologic pregnancies. The arrows in the lower portion of the diagram indicate the direction; the values assigned to them, the hourly transfer in milliliters. The heavy circles to the left of each diagram designate the direction of the net transfer, in other words, the "circulation" of the water. (From D. L. Hutchinson et al.[1])

In early gestation (12 weeks) the exchange of water between the amniotic fluid and the mother is of about the same magnitude as the exchange between mother and fetus, as shown in Fig. 2.3. The exchange between fetus and amniotic fluid is small by comparison. The role of the fetus in the transfer of amniotic fluid becomes more significant as pregnancy advances. At term about 40 percent of the water transfer from amniotic fluid to mother is accomplished through the intermedium of the fetus. The role of the fetus in the various exchange mechanisms thus changes as term approaches.

The site and mechanisms responsible for water exchange between the mother and amniotic fluid have not yet been identified, and direct exchange through the placental membrane and decidua cannot be excluded. The Hutchinson group proposed that, because of the high concentration of tritium found in Wharton's jelly, a major part of water exchange of the amniotic fluid may take place through this organ. The mechanisms and site of exchanges between amniotic fluid and the fetus are also not entirely clear, but fetal urination and swallowing of amniotic fluid seem to be major factors of importance.

The exchanges occurring between the fetus and amniotic fluid and amniotic fluid and the mother can become more important in the presence of placental dysfunction. Hutchinson and his co-workers[7] found in the pathologic condition of hydramnios, which they investigated in two cases in a similar manner, that the rate of water exchange directly between the maternal and fetal membranes was grossly impaired. In the presence of hydramnios the exchange rate between mother and fetus (placental) was reduced considerably below that found in normal pregnant women and the transfer from the amniotic fluid directly to the mother was proportionally increased (Fig. 2.3). Surprisingly, the total amount of water leaving the amniotic fluid was not appreciably different in the two conditions. The rate of "removal" of water from the amniotic cavity was not decreased; if anything it was increased. The important difference in hydramnios lay in the bypass of the fetus as the major intermedium of exchange between amniotic fluid and the mother. The mechanism is unknown but could reflect a lesion of the fetoplacentary circulatory system. The data reveal that changes in alternate routes of exchange occur when actual exchange of water between the mother and fetus is greatly depressed.

Quantitative measurements of exchange rates for sodium and potassium have been made in primates and the data indicate that each constituent is exchanged at its own characteristic rate, indicating the complexities of the exchange mechanisms involved.[47] Exchange rates of some metabolites (lactic acid and urea, for example) have also been studied in primates. These are more complicated to analyze since they can be metabolized by mother or fetus as well as exchanged.

Hutchinson and his associates,[52] in a most important study of urea (the major end product of nitrogen metabolism in the fetus), have shown that there is a rapid exchange of C^{14}-labeled urea in primates between maternal and fetal blood and an appreciably slower transfer involving amniotic fluid. Urea in the amniotic fluid was derived from both the mother and the fetus in an approximate ratio of 3:1. The endogenous urea production of the fetus was estimated to account for less than one-tenth of the total placental exchange. The exchange of urea in the amniotic fluid proceeds equally rapidly when the fetus has been subjected to nephrectomy in utero. The rate of excretion of urea by the fetal kidney in utero thus is clearly not dependent solely on the rate of fetal production of urea, nor is fetal urine the only source for urea found in the amniotic fluid.

We are now accumulating a most important body of new information defining the complex pathways whereby placental exchange normally maintains fetal and maternal plasma pH and concentrations of solute, sodium, chloride, HCO_3, urea, and creatinine in equilibrium. In this situation the fetal kidney appears to be operating physiologically, albeit in a passive subordinate capacity since fetal renal function is not essential for maintenance of fetal life in utero. Fetal renal function does, however, influence the volume and composition of amniotic fluid, and the changes observed in it during gestation warrant consideration.

CHANGES IN VOLUME AND COMPOSITION OF AMNIOTIC FLUID DURING GESTATION

Amniotic fluid resembles fetal urine more closely than fetal plasma in most respects.[3,14] The concentration of nonprotein nitrogenous compounds in amniotic fluid (urea, uric acid, and creatinine) rises above that in fetal plasma after the first trimester and keeps increasing up to term, as shown in Table 2.4. The total volume of amniotic fluid varies considerably. No measurements are available before 10 weeks, but considerable data are now available[50,53,54] after this time up to delivery. The volume of amniotic fluid is about 30 ml at 10 weeks.[54] The rate

TABLE 2.4   Changes in amniotic fluid volume, osmolality, and creatinine
concentration with advancing pregnancy

Gestational age (weeks)	Volume[a] (ml)		Osmolality[b] (mOsm/l)		Creatinine[c] (mg%)	
	Mean	Range	Mean	Range	Mean	Range
10	30	(29–32)				
20	302	(270–340)	263	(256–269)	0.87	(0.8–1.0)
30			259	(225–269)	1.14	(0.9–1.3)
37	687	(229–1,338)	252	(249–255)		
38	1032	(553–1,512)			2.03	(1.5–2.7)
40	791	(330–1,455)	246	(240–250)		
42	324	(0–441)	242	(240–243)	2.78	(2.5–3.0)

[a] A. E. Seeds, Jr.[50] and P. N. Gillibrand.[54]
[b] P. A. Miles and J. W. Pearson.[58]
[c] R. M. Pitkin and S. J. Zwirek.[57]

of increase is more rapid after 14 to 15 weeks,[53] suggesting that fetal
micturition may be contributing significantly from this time on. The volume then increases to a maximal volume of about 1,000 ml at 38 weeks,
after which it progressively and rapidly declines as pregnancy continues.

Gillibrand[55] has measured the rate of water transfer from the amniotic
sac during advancing pregnancy by the use of deuterium oxide. He found
that the rate of water transfer from the amniotic sac increases less rapidly
than volume with advancing pregnancy and it decreases with post-
maturity. The transfer rate of water is independent of amniotic fluid
volume at all stages of pregnancy. The maturity of the fetus appears
to influence water transfer rates from the amniotic sac, possibly because
of decreasing absorption by fetal skin as cornification occurs. The health
of the fetus is an important factor influencing amniotic fluid volume,
large volumes being found when the fetus is abnormal (as in anencephaly
and duodenal atresia) and low volumes with fetal death.[56] The decrease
in amniotic fluid volume noted after 37 to 38 weeks of gestation coincides
with the time when creatinine is rising most rapidly in the amniotic
fluid.

Pitkin and Zwirek's data[57] showed that a gradual increase in creatinine
concentration occurs from 10 to 15 weeks up to about the thirty-fourth
week, after which there is a more abrupt rise (see Table 2.4). After
37 weeks creatinine is present in amniotic fluid in a concentration two
to three times the normal maternal serum level. These authors proposed

that the presence of creatinine in amniotic fluid in concentrations of 2 mg percent or higher might be clinically useful as an index of fetal maturity. While the rise in creatinine concentration near the end of the pregnancy could be explained by the diminution in amniotic fluid volume, this is presently speculation and additional factors may be involved.

As indicated in Table 2.4, the osmolality of amniotic fluid is close to but slightly less than that of fetal and maternal serum in the first trimester and gradually decreases reaching the lowest values in the last trimester. Miles and Pearson[58] consider values below 250 mOsm/l as evidence of fetal maturity. The values for osmolality continue to decrease in pregnancies going beyond 39 to 40 weeks despite the progressive oligohydramnios that is seen in this condition indicating decreased rates for transfer of water out of the amniotic sac.

Less is known about other constituents. The protein concentration is low (0.22 to 0.31 gm percent), but the percentage of albumin and α, β, and γ globulins resembles that of fetal serum except for being relatively free of lipoproteins and fibrinogen. The electrolyte composition of amniotic fluid resembles fetal extracellular fluid in that the concentrations of sodium, chloride, and carbon dioxide are high and only small amounts of potassium, calcium, phosphate, and magnesium are present.[14,47] The composition of human amniotic fluid is now being intensively studied and current monographs cover the subject quite completely.[47,59]

CIRCULATION OF THE AMNIOTIC FLUID

The amniotic fluid has been thought of as a stagnant pool, but it is actually a fluid in dynamic though slow equilibrium with its surroundings. Recent studies in primates have revealed the main pathways of what can be best termed the "circulation" of this vital fluid.[47] While the quantitative aspects of influx (formation) and efflux (removal) of amniotic fluid in man have yet to be accurately documented, we can make certain general statements. Fetal urination and absorption by other organs (such as the lungs, skin, and gut) and their secretions contribute to the formation and composition of the amniotic fluid. The fetus provides a major route for its removal. Clinical observations bear out the participation of the fetus in the circulation of this fluid. Oligohydramnios is commonly encountered in association with obstruction to urinary outflow or renal agenesis, and hydramnios is frequently found when fetal deglutition is not possible.[46,60] Polyhydramnios has been associated with pregnancies resulting in the birth of infants with nephrogenic diabetes insipidus[61] and congenital chloridorrhea, a congenital form of chronic diarrhea[62] resulting from faulty resorption of chloride by the gut.

While the water exchange occurring directly between the amniotic fluid and the mother may be greater than that occurring with the fetus as an intermedium, the quantity of amniotic fluid exchanged with the fetus (by fetal turnover via urination into and ingestion and absorption of amniotic fluid by the fetus) appears to be substantial. Pritchard[63] has shown, in an ingeniously designed study, that the fetus at term swallows or otherwise absorbs about 20 ml of amnioic fluid/hour or nearly 500 ml/day. This would represent a substantial daily fluid intake for a full-term fetus. Pritchard cited the coincidence between the values for the rate of fetal urination of rhesus monkeys at term reported by Chez, Smith, and Hutchinson[64] to average 5 ml/kg/hr and his data on human fetal deglutition which averaged out to 5 ml/kg/hr. Fetal urination and deglutition are probably functionally related. Since the amniotic fluid is hypotonic, its daily ingestion by the fetus in these quantities would be sufficient to account for the persistent hypotonicity of fetal urine. An infant ingesting this volume of hypotonic amniotic fluid would have no need to concentrate his urine to conserve water. A mild water diuresis would be the only appropriate renal response.

It is of interest that McCance and Widdowson's data[17] given in Table 2.1 show that a prompt elevation in urine solute concentration was observed in all of the infants they studied in the first 24 hours after their removal from the uterine environment by normal delivery. The "physiologic dehydration" of these newborns thus became evident when they could no longer imbibe amniotic fluid. While the fetal kidney can excrete a hypertonic urine, it does not appear to do so normally in utero. This seemingly paradoxical situation may not be unphysiologic or inappropriate to the fetal environment in utero as previously thought, since the fetal kidney may be responding—appropriately—to the fetal imbibition of (hypotonic) amniotic fluid.

SUMMARY

The available data provide direct evidence that the initial step in urine formation in the fetal metanephric kidney—glomerular ultrafiltration—occurs in a manner qualitatively similar to that of the adult kidney.

The alterations found in composition of fetal urine as compared to plasma indicate that tubular resorption of filtered solutes is also qualitatively similar. In view of the evidence that the bulk of filtered sodium, chloride, and bicarbonate is resorbed, it seems reasonable to assume that the resorption of the major ions of the extracellular fluid involves the same active "threshold" and carrier exchange transport mechanisms (sodium and chloride resorption and secretion of hydrogen and/or potassium and organic acid anions) that operate in the kidney of the newborn and adult. There is little quantitative data available regarding the more or less discrete Tm-limited resorptive mechanism (phosphate, glucose, amino acids, uric acid, and so forth). The virtual absence of glucose and phosphate from fetal urine when they are present in the fetal plasma ultrafiltrate demonstrates that these two discrete transport mechanisms are functional in the fetal kidney.

The higher concentration of urea and creatinine in urine than in fetal plasma supports the idea that passive diffusion serves to achieve osmolar equilibrium of water and solute between the tubular lumen and peritubular capillaries in the immature nephrons just as it does in the mature kidney. The elaboration by the fetal kidney of a *hypo*tonic urine implies that the loop of Henle becomes functionally active in utero, as does the evidence that a *hyper*tonic urine can be elaborated under certain conditions by the fetus.

The reliance on data in other mammals for a description of the pattern of functional maturation of the kidney in man is obviously hazardous. The kidneys of mammals at the time of birth vary in different species with respect to their morphologic and functional development. All newborn animals do not have kidneys of similar maturity. One of the most obvious differences is between the rat and man. The rat develops two-thirds of its nephrons after birth, while no new nephrons form postnatally in man. It is important to keep these species variations in mind, especially since some of the maturation phenomena could well occur at different times in different species and extrapolation of the results of one species to another could be misleading.

One possible generalization is that the data reviewed do indicate that the maturing kidney is not only growing but functioning in utero, achieving a surprising degree of sophistication by the time of birth. The fetal kidney is apparently a passive observer with respect to its lack of responsibility for regulatory functions in the fetal environment. It is nonetheless participating very actively as a functioning kidney. While this is teleologically comforting when we consider the "work load" that lies ahead at the moment of birth, viewed in developmental terms it also means that the uterine environment has actually allowed an essential first stage of a continuing maturation process to be completed.

Further studies of kidney development are needed if we are to describe the functional correlates of this early in-utero growth and maturation. It is clearly more than a stage of embryogenesis, because organ differentiation also occurs. It is of interest that the fetal internal environment during this first phase of renal functional maturation is uniquely monitored by placental function. This period of equilibrium contrasts with the succeeding one, in which great stress will be placed on the kidney to function as a kidney as soon as extrauterine life begins. While the growth process postnatally involves new physiologic stresses, this does not necessarily mean that different factors are operating to stimulate growth and regulate function. It seems likely that the same factors acting after growth has ceased in the adult to maintain glomerotubular balance also operate in utero and postnatally.

Fetal and neonatal animals provide a unique developmental model for study of the appropriateness of observed or induced phenomena when related to the environmental situation normally experienced by the immature subject. Too often the unique environmental aspects have received little attention in the interpretation of observations by the investigator. Interpretation has dealt instead with a comparative analysis of the results (usually in inappropriate quantitative terms) against results obtained in comparable experimental circumstances but in stable nongrowing adults.

Hopefully, future studies will also provide data useful in defining functional relationships in individual but representative immature as well as mature nephrons. We shall then be able to characterize the differences in individual nephron function, as well as in total organ function, that occur with maturation.

It is important to realize that the fetal kidney may respond to drugs and hormones administered to the mother when these substances cross the placenta in a biologically active form. Maternal polyhydramnios and neonatal hyponatremia have been observed by the author in association with the prolonged maternal ingestion of the naturetic chlorothiazide. The fetal kidney may well have participated in the evolution of this disturbance in fetal and placental sodium and water balance. Consideration should thus be given to the possible effects on fetal kidney function of drugs given for their renal effects in the mother.

Chapter 3. Quantitative Measurement of Renal Function during Growth in Infancy and Childhood

The period from birth to maturity is one in which growth is continuously present but is proceeding at varying rates. Consequently increases in absolute values for all discrete renal functions will occur throughout childhood growth. The most direct way to assess "normality" of the achievement of renal function in growing subjects at a given age would be to compare actual measurements for the parameters of concern in a specific patient with a centile for that function derived from serial studies of similar measurements obtained from adequate samples of normal subjects of comparable age. This could be done most directly by the construction of standard regression curves based on measured actual values for the various parameters from infancy to adolescence. Unfortunately, present data are not adequate for this purpose.

The absence of such standards for assessment of the adequacy of various aspects of renal function in a particular infant or child poses problems for the clinician and the investigator. Postmortem studies have demonstrated that there is a good correlation between renal weight and both age and height during childhood.[1,2] Radiographic measurements of kidney length and cross-sectional area have also been demonstrated to correlate closely with age and height and weight.[3,4] The use of size alone (determined directly or radiologically) is, however, too crude an index of function to define normal or abnormal function. The finding of small-sized but normally formed kidneys in a small child offers information of limited value if one is interested in defining possible causal relationships that may exist between the two. Until we can determine the total number of individual functioning nephrons, the only alternative approach is quantitative measurement of overall renal function by discrete parameters.

The earlier studies of the relation between kidney function and size during growth were performed in animals.[5] Increases in renal functional capacity have now been shown to parallel the increases in kidney weight and in body size occurring with growth in many mammals, but meaningful correlations between these various parameters during the different periods of growth from fetal life to postpuberty have yet to be established.[6] Smith's development of renal clearance techniques[7] has provided the means for directly partitioning renal function in man into three discrete measurable components. The values for each component may vary directly with body size in adults and are quantitatively reproducible in any one subject who is in a steady state.

These three components are glomerular filtration rate (GFR), renal blood flow (RBF), and tubular transport capacity for p-aminohippurate (Tm_{PAH}) and glucose ($Tm_{GLUCOSE}$). Measurements of these parameters in infants and children at different ages have provided data that can be used to quantitate changes in renal function associated with growth. Interrelationships between these functions can also be defined to characterize components of renal function with respect to overall values for filtration fraction, blood flow per unit of tubular mass, and filtration per gram of tubular mass during growth.

The method most commonly employed to measure GFR is inulin clearance (C_{IN}), which has been shown to be an accurate means of measuring GFR in infants and adults.[7,8,9] The measurement of C_{IN} requires intravenous administration of a priming dose of inulin followed by constant infusion to maintain stable blood levels, and the collection of serial accurately timed urine samples usually by indwelling catheter. The mean value obtained by measurement of the endogenous creatinine clearance (C_{CR}) correlates well with the simultaneously measured C_{IN}, but the large standard error (± 18.7 percent) for the value of GFR measured by C_{CR} in individual periods precludes its use alone when a more accurate estimate of GFR is desired.[10]

The feasibility of using radioactively tagged substances for standard clearance measurements after a single injection to measure GFR with and without collection of bladder urine is being explored in children.[10,11] At the present time the results of clearance measurements comparing inulin with sodium iothalamate I^{131} indicate that the latter gives values comparable to C_{IN} when urine collections are made. A comparative study made by Cohen and his fellow investigators[10] showed an excellent correlation ($r = 0.987$) between simultaneously measured clearance by inulin and sodium iothalamate I^{131}. The former was given as a priming dose and sustained by constant infusion; the latter was given as a single injection. Patients were hydrated, following which three urine collections were obtained by voluntary voiding.

The usefulness of clearances utilizing sodium iothalamate I^{131} administered in a single injection without urine collection is limited since the method then appears to give values for GFR that approximate, in reliability, those measured by endogenous creatinine clearance.[11] On the basis of presently available evidence single injection methods without urine collection thus do not provide accuracy of quantitative measurement of GFR in infants and children comparable to standard techniques relying on urine collection. For a discussion of the theoretic basis of single injection procedures and their advantages and limitations in pediatrics the interested reader should consult the literature.[10–14]

Renal blood flow can be measured by determining the clearance of any substance whose rate of extraction from the renal arterial blood in one circulation through the kidney is known. The method most frequently employed to measure renal blood flow in man has been the measurement of the clearance of p-aminohippurate (C_{PAH}). At low plasma concentrations (2 to 10 mg percent) C_{PAH} can be used as an estimate of effective renal plasma flow (RPF) because it has been shown that about 90 percent of the free "unbound" PAH in blood is removed in one circulation through the kidney under these conditions. Renal blood flow is the product[7] of C_{PAH} (representing RPF) $\times$ I (I/HCT). Renal arteriovenous (A-V) extraction of PAH in man normally averages about 91 percent. True renal plasma flow thus exceeds C_{PAH} by 9 percent. However, C_{PAH} may not provide an approximation of true renal plasma flow in the diseased kidney because the A-V extraction ratio progressively declines with parenchymal damage or destruction.

One factor accounting for incomplete extraction of PAH is protein binding. Protein binding of PAH in plasma ranges from 10 to 20 percent. The rate of filtration of PAH is a linear function of the concentration of the free unbound moiety in plasma.[15] The blood perfusing nonexcretory tissues (that is, the renal capsule, perirenal fat, and pelvis) also contributes to a lowered extraction ratio. Removal of PAH is accomplished by both glomerular filtration and tubular secretion. Since PAH is secreted only by the proximal tubules, that portion of blood perfusing the medulla and papillae flowing through the vasa recta from juxtamedullary efferent arterioles has a lower extraction ratio because PAH is then removed only by filtration.[15] It is estimated that most of the renal blood flow perfuses the cortical nephrons; the juxtamedullary nephrons and medulla receive only about one-fifth of total renal blood flow in adult man. The intrarenal distribution of blood flow in the mature kidney is not, however, rigidly fixed.

Knowledge of the distribution of renal blood flow is as important in understanding the overall functional state of the kidney as information about the rate of renal blood flow. A detailed analysis of the renal circulation and the variety of tubular-vascular arrangements present has recently been presented by Barger and Herd[16] along with a review of the methods for measuring the intrarenal distribution of blood flow. The most widely used method for measurement of distribution of renal blood flow in man is the inert gas "washout" technique originally introduced for animal studies by Thorburn and his co-workers,[17] utilizing the renal arterial injection of a bolus of saline saturated with radioactive krypton (85_{Kr}) or xenon (133_{Xe}).

Four components with different flow rates have been identified by analysis of disappearance curves of radioactive isotopes, monitored by an external detector. These have been localized in the dog by autoradiographs and shown to represent rates of flow through (1) the cortex; (2) the inner or juxtamedullary cortex and outer medulla; (3) the vasa recta and inner medulla, and (4) the perirenal and hilar fat. In man the localization is less precise but two compartments can be identified, a rapid-filling one representing outer cortical vascular filling and a second component representing juxtamedullary cortical and outer-medullary vascular density. In normal human subjects the cortex receives three-fourths of the total renal blood flow, with a flow rate of about 400 ml per 100 grams of cortex per minute. The juxtamedullary cortex and outer medulla receive a fifth of the flow at a slower rate of about 125 ml/100 grams/minute.[16]

The rate of salt and water excretion may be profoundly altered in the normal kidney by changes in distribution of blood flow and filtration produced by increases or decreases in fluid volumes of the body. Active tubular resorption of sodium may itself be modified as a result of alterations in the forces affecting passive capillary uptake of resorption. Direct evidence supporting this hypothesis was first obtained by Windhager,

Lewy, and Spitzer,[18] who demonstrated that an increase in the colloid osmotic pressure in superficial peritubular capillaries in the rat facilitates proximal tubular resorption of sodium and water, whereas an increase in hydrostatic pressure depresses resorption.

In the superficial cortical nephrons of the mature mammalian kidney where peritubular capillaries connect in series with glomerular capillaries of the same nephron, changes in rate of glomerular blood flow or filtration have predictable effects on peritubular capillary hydrostatic and plasma colloid osmotic forces.

In juxtamedullary nephrons the arrangement is more complex, partly because of differences in the blood supply to the proximal tubules and that forming the vasa recta. In addition, the blood flow through juxtamedullary nephrons is extremely variable, further complicating the description of the resorptive process in the juxtamedullary cortex and outer medulla. The flow in these two compartments has been shown to vary under certain physiologic conditions in man,[19] in the dog,[20] and in the rat.[21] The proportion of total RBF through these two compartments in the immature kidney is not known and may well differ from that found after dimensional differences between outer and inner cortical nephrons present at birth have disappeared. A greater proportional flow to compartment 2, the deeper (juxtamedullary) nephrons, than to compartment 1, the outer cortex, might be expected in the kidney of the newborn because of the more advanced development and size of juxtamedullary nephrons relative to the outer cortical nephrons.[22]

One of the difficulties faced in evaluating studies of RPF in the infant is that the value of C_{PAH} is not an accurate measure of total renal plasma flow until after 6 months of age. Calcagno and Rubin[23] found the value for renal extraction of PAH (E_{PAH}) to be low (average 58.6 percent) in four infants studied between 8 days and 3 months of age, while values for infants 5 months of age and older approximated the value for E_{PAH} found in adults (93.5 percent). Accordingly the true minimal effective renal blood flow in infants less than 6 months old is higher than that calculated from C_{PAH} and the E_{PAH} is probably lowest in the newborn. A similar situation has been described (that is, low values for E_{PAH} in comparison to adult values in the newborn) in the young rat[24] and dog.[25] The extraction of PAH rises with increasing postnatal age in both animals, reaching mature value at about 18 days of age in the rat and about 10 weeks after birth in the dog.

The factors responsible for depressed PAH extraction by the infant kidney would include: (1) greater diversion of blood flow away from nephrons (nutrient blood flow); (2) diversion of a greater proportion of renal blood flow to juxtamedullary nephrons than to outer cortical nephrons; and (3) reduced proximal tubular excretory capacity for PAH arising from immaturity of the proximal tubules or reduced tubular mass relative to glomerular area.

If forces regulating glomerular filtration are similar in the infant and adult kidney, the finding of slightly higher values for inulin extraction ratios (24 percent) in infants under 6 months than in adults (20 percent) by Calcagno and Rubin would not support the first factor as being significant. The filtration fraction ($FF = C_{IN}/C_{PAH}$) will also be inaccurate as long as E_{PAH} is reduced. In the studies of Horster and Lewy on young rats[24] and of Horster and Valtin on puppies[25] the true FF was measured (C_{PAH}/E_{PAH}) and found to be less than that in the mature animal in both subjects at birth, rising to the mature value at approximately the same time as E_{PAH} reached the mature value. This was interpreted as evidence reflecting the existence of significant nutrient blood flow to developing hypofunctional glomeruli and nephrons in the kidney in the neonatal period. The data of Calcagno and Rubin on E_{PAH} in small infants suggests that the FF would be at least 30 percent lower than the value given by C_{IN}/C_{PAH} and that the true FF might also be less than 0.20 (mature value), but data are not adequate to determine how the true FF in the newborn infant compares with the adult.

One possibility raised by Calcagno and Rubin to explain the lower extraction ratio for PAH was that in the infant kidney a greater proportion of intrarenal blood flow might pass to deep (juxtamedullary) nephrons than to the less anatomically developed cortical nephrons. Recent studies[26] of the intrarenal distribution of blood flow in the kidneys of young puppies have shown that the proportion going to superficial (cortical) nephrons in 6-week-old puppies is lower than in 16-week-old puppies. The lower cortical flow was also associated with a lower value for E_{PAH}—0.44, which had risen to 0.75 at 16 weeks (normal for mature dogs). These data provide the first direct evidence suggesting that the distribution of intrarenal blood flow to outer and inner cortex in the immature kidney may differ from that found in the mature subject. A major factor accounting for reduced E_{PAH} is the reduced secretory and resorptive transport capacity of the proximal tubules in the immature nephrons. This aspect is described more fully later in this chapter.

The values of the maximal rate (tubular capacity) for secretion of

PAH (Tm_{PAH}) are useful to measure the overall capacity of tubular mechanisms for transport of special materials from peritubular fluid to tubular lumen. This provides the most direct quantitative measurement of overall functioning tubular mass. Tubular secretion resembles tubular resorption in many respects—the major difference being one of orientation of the transport mechanism.[27] If maximal tubular transport capacity is to be used as a measure of active functioning tubular mass, the system employed must involve an active secretory mechanism which exhibits an absolute limitation of transport capacity for which the term Tm (tubular maxima) is applied to indicate a Tm/transport-limited mechanism.

One Tm-limited mechanism is PAH secretion. Glucose resorption is also a Tm-limited mechanism and values for $Tm_{GLUCOSE}$ are useful to measure functioning tubular mass in the normal[28,29] and the diseased kidney.[30] The values for $Tm_{GLUCOSE}$ vary in a parallel manner with those for Tm_{PAH} when changes occur in overall tubular transport associated with normal growth, with compensatory hypertrophy, or with physiologic alterations of blood or energy supply to the proximal tubules. When these three aspects of renal function are measured simultaneously, the composite function of the normal kidney can be quantitated and the interrelations between glomerular filtration and renal blood flow and tubular activity can be defined. New information has become available in the last two decades by application of quantitative clearance techniques to children, describing changes that occur in renal function during certain periods of growth in childhood.[31-35] These data have also been used to compare certain aspects of function in infants and adults.[8,36,37]

THE KIDNEY AT BIRTH

Anatomic Characteristics

It has long been recognized that the human kidney at birth is anatomically distinguishable from the mature organ by gross morphology and microscopic histologic criteria. Even though nephron induction normally ceases before term (the thirty-sixth week of gestation) the last nephrons induced (which are confined to the subcapsular region of the cortex) may still be recognizable in early infancy by their immaturity. Anatomic classification of developmental age based on graded signs of "nephrogenic activity" has been defined.[38,39] The major indication of persistent nephrogenic activity consists in the finding of primitive nephrons characterized by their heavily cellular primitive S-shape or rudimentary glomerular tufts that lack a true vascular pole. The kidney of the normal full-term (38 weeks) newborn shows little if any evidence of such immaturity.

The amount of nephrogenic activity present in the cortex has been used by Potter and Thierstein[38] as an anatomic index of gestational age. Macdonald and Emery[39] in a recent study of normal newborns did not find any truly "primitive" glomeruli present in kidneys in infants after the forty-fourth week of gestation. The correlation of signs of glomerular maturity with body length was less than that found with age. The glomerular maturity of low-birth-weight-for-age infants (fetal malnutrition) thus correlates with gestational age rather than weight. They concluded that the persistence of primitive glomeruli beyond the forty-fourth week of gestation can be considered as evidence of abnormal or delayed renal maturation.

The kidney continues to increase in mass postnatally by active cellular growth primarily involving the outer medulla and cortex. The size of all parts of the nephrons increases. The changes in size and configuration of the individual nephrons during normal postnatal development have, however, only recently been studied in a comprehensive manner. Quantitative data of this type documenting the diversity in dimensions of the nephrons found in the normal immature kidney are essential if correlations between structure and function are to be sought during renal development. Such information is also necessary to provide a background to standardize the range of normal dimensions characterizing the different ages of development from infancy through adolescence before abnormal dimensions indicative of disease can be firmly established.

The anatomic dimensions and characteristics of the nephrons in the kidney at birth are quite different than those in the adult. The morphologic changes during maturation have been well documented in careful studies by Fetterman and his associates.[22] His group compared various dimensions of glomeruli and proximal tubules isolated by microdissection from kidneys of subjects varying in age from newborn to 18 years. Their most striking finding in the kidney of the newborn was the physical underdevelopment of the proximal tubules relative to their corresponding glomeruli. The mean glomerular diameter in the newborn is about 0.11 mm, about one-third that of the adult (0.28 mm), as shown in Table 3.1. The mean length of proximal tubules, however, is about 2 mm, or one-tenth that of the adult (20 mm).

Nephron heterogeneity (variation in size between individual nephrons

TABLE 3.1 Mean glomerular diameter and proximal length for three cortical levels (designated as outer, middle, inner) of nephrons in twenty-three cases studied (from G. H. Fetterman et al.[22])

Series no.	Age	Mean glomerular diameter (mm)			Mean proximal length (mm)		
		Outer	Middle	Inner	Outer	Middle	Inner
MD 6	Term	0.106	0.115	0.129	1.26	1.73	2.46
CA-7-60	1 month	0.105	0.109	0.123	2.29	2.94	3.37
CA-12-57	3½ months	0.101	0.125	0.142	2.83	3.19	4.12
MD 52	5 months	0.155	0.151	0.163	6.54	6.78	7.17
CA-62-59	6 months	0.150	0.165	0.184	4.84	6.05	6.74
MD 81	11 months	0.122	0.122	0.131	4.87	4.70	4.86
CA-93-62	12 months	0.124	0.117	0.132	6.38	6.01	6.37
CA-5-60	14 months	0.168	0.168	0.173	7.16	7.98	7.86
MD 25	20 months	0.152	0.157	0.158	5.52	5.74	5.39
CA-4-59	22 months	0.175	0.175	0.174	7.53	8.52	8.36
CA-14-60	27 months	0.175	0.162	0.186	7.99	8.24	8.51
CA-148-63	3 years	0.170	0.164	0.176	8.03	8.24	6.99
MD 50	3 years	0.169	0.166	0.181	7.37	7.28	7.82
MD 23	3½ years	0.178	0.178	0.188	6.29	7.14	7.50
MD 41	3½ years	0.201	0.201	0.200	8.61	9.15	8.17
MD 58	5 years	0.146	0.155	0.154	7.05	6.93	6.91
CA-56-59	6 years	0.190	0.204	0.212	8.34	9.92	9.51
CA-111-59	7½ years	0.215	0.221	0.230	10.72	10.94	12.91
CA-183-58	8½ years	0.192	0.196	0.204	12.29	13.73	13.82
MD 28	12 years	0.241	0.249	0.249	11.74	11.95	12.70
MD 21	13 years	0.243	0.235	0.237	12.72	13.06	12.84
MD 38	15 years	0.222	0.212	0.229	15.21	12.99	13.47
MD 40	18 years	0.196	0.207	0.197	11.68	12.78	11.53
Composite adult kidney	35 years (average)	0.287	0.280	0.283	21.5	19.4	17.8

from the same level of the cortex of the kidney) was another striking finding in the newborn kidney. Heterogeneity was evident in the great variation (elevenfold) noted between lengths of the shortest and longest proximal tubules in the infant cortex, in contrast to the small (twofold) variation characteristic of the mature kidney. While the glomeruli also showed individual variation in size, they were much more uniform in the newborn kidney.

In addition, the dimensions of glomeruli and nephrons in the outer cortex proved to be smaller than those in the inner cortex. The mean glomerular diameters in the three levels of the cortex in the newborn kidney were as follows (see Table 3.1): outer, 0.106 mm; middle, 0.115 mm; and inner, 0.129 mm. The mean length of proximal tubules varied in the same direction: 1.26 mm, outer; 1.73 mm, middle; and 2.46 mm, inner. These variations are caused by differences in maturation (developmental age) of nephrons. The oldest nephrons are most mature and largest and are found in the deeper cortex in the juxtamedullary area.

These differences in glomerular size in the different levels of the immature cortex contrast with the findings in the mature kidney, where mean glomerular diameter is about the same in all levels and the longest proximal tubules are found on nephrons occupying the outer cortex (Table 3.1). The dimensional differences in mean glomerular diameter in outer and inner levels of the kidney of the newborn are of a sufficient order of magnitude that one might expect a significant difference in single nephron GFR in the two levels of the cortex, the higher value to be found in the deeper nephrons. The expectation, based on the anatomic evidence, that there would be such functional differences is supported by a recent report[40] employing micropuncture to measure single nephron GFR in the young rat. It was found that GFR could be as much as 50 percent greater in deeper nephrons than in superficial nephrons.

Fetterman and his associates[22] found that these dimensional variations between nephrons in different levels of the cortex disappear in man by 12 to 14 months of age. The tubules thus appear to grow more rapidly than the glomeruli during this period of early postnatal growth, since the mean glomerular diameter at this age has increased only slightly (0.14) while the mean proximal tubular length has more than tripled (6.9 mm) in comparison to the respective values in the newborn kidney.

The individual glomeruli and their respective tubules are, however, generally well matched for size in the newborn kidney in spite of the variations described. The smallest (and most immature) glomeruli are found in the outer cortex and have the shortest and least coiled proximal tubules, while the largest (and most mature) glomeruli lying in the inner levels have the longest and most highly coiled proximal tubules. This finding indicates that individual nephron growth during organogenesis appears to be generally allometric, thus preserving balance with respect to the physical dimensions of individual glomeruli and their attached renal tubules. The growth of nephrons in the early postnatal period serves two developmental purposes. It corrects heterogeneity reflecting differences in nephron maturation and age and it increases tubular size more than glomerular size thus achieving better anatomic glomerular balance than exists at the time of birth.

Changes in Renal Function in the Neonatal Period

Birth is associated with the requirement for profound changes in organ function essential to sustain homeostasis appropriate to the newly assumed biologic independence of the infant from its mother. There are pronounced circulatory adjustments that occur upon removal of the placenta as a regulator of the infant's internal milieu. The circulatory changes involving the lungs and heart are well recognized but those involving parenchymal organs such as the liver and kidneys are less well known. Cineangiography in the human infant in utero[41] has shown that substantial quantities of umbilical vein blood pass through the ductus venosum and bypass the substance of the liver. The ductus venosum closes after birth and portal blood flow to the liver increases markedly. Some enzymes suddenly increase greatly in activity and others decrease. Rappaport[42] has suggested that such functional alterations may relate to the marked changes occurring in intrahepatic circulation creating a new circulatory milieu. The changes in renal circulation at birth in lambs were described in Chapter 2. There is direct evidence that similar changes occur in the human in the first few days of neonatal life.

Oh, Oh, and Lind[43] measured GFR (C_{IN}) and RPF (C_{PAH}) in a group of normal newborns immediately after birth and again at 2 to 5 days of age (see Table 3.2). The mean values for C_{IN} and C_{PAH}

TABLE 3.2   Renal function in newborn infants with early and late cord clamping (from W. Oh, M. A. Oh, and J. Lind[43])

Age group	1–12 hours			2–5 days		
	Early clamped	Late clamped	P	Early clamped	Late clamped	P
GFR (C_{IN}) in ml/min/1.73 m² S.A.	20.3 ±1.2	28.6 ±1.9	<.001	33.0 ±3.6	37.5 ±4.1	>.05
C_{PAH} in ml/min/ 1.73 m² S.A.	71.0 ±3.8	96.0 ±4.4	<.001	129.0 ±15.0	136.0 ±14.0	>.05
Filtration fraction	0.31 ±0.03	0.31 ±0.02	>.05	0.27 ±0.03	0.30 ±0.03	>.05
Number of infants	14	29		8	18	

per 1.73 m² S.A. had increased by 40 and 50 percent respectively by the third day. These investigators also found that mean values at birth for C_{IN} and C_{PAH} were higher in infants with late cord clamping as compared to early clamping, but these differences disappeared by 3 days of age. Even though true RBF in the newborn infant is not accurately measured by C_{PAH}, the change in values indicates that an abrupt increase in RBF occurs in the neonatal period.

Actual values for discrete renal functions at birth are related to both body size and gestational age. Values for GFR and C_{PAH} are generally lower in low-weight (usually also prematurely born) infants than in normal-weight, full-term infants. Furthermore, there is evidence that the postnatal increase that occurs is independent of gestational age. Barnett and his co-workers[31] found values for GFR, RPF, and Tm_{PAH} determined in a group of premature infants when they were 2 to 3 months of postnatal age and had achieved a mean weight of 2.4 kg that were 36 to 58 percent higher than those found in a group of 3- to 13-day-old premature infants whose mean weight was similar (2.2 kg) at the time of study and who would be considered to be of approximately comparable gestational age if judged by weight.

The animal studies of fetal and perinatal circulation cited in Chapter 2 provide a partial explanation for the rapid increase seen in renal function in the immediate postnatal period. Since the fetal kidney plays a relatively passive functional role in regulation of the composition and volume of fetal body fluids, it is not surprising that it receives a diminished blood supply. The circulatory adjustments at birth are probably only one factor influencing GFR and renal blood flow. The removal of the placenta places a new functional load on the kidney of the newborn at the time of birth. These two factors provide a new growth stimulus in the neonatal period, but additional mechanisms may also be responsible for the rapid increases in renal function that occur.

CHANGES IN RENAL FUNCTION OCCURRING WITH CHILDHOOD GROWTH

A major difficulty faced by anyone attempting to define a pattern underlying the observed changes in renal function during the period of childhood growth is the scarcity of data on subjects beyond infancy in later childhood. The great majority of reported studies of renal function in normal pediatric subjects have been made in normal neonates or prematurely born infants who remain institutionalized until they achieve weights of 2 kg or greater, by which time they are 2 to 3 months of age. There is only one report in the literature describing a large number of simultaneous measurements of GFR, RPF or C_{PAH}, and Tm_{PAH} in presumably normal children older than 6 months. This study by Rubin, Bruck, and Rapoport[32] includes forty-one children between 6 months and 12 years of age. These authors used mannitol for estimation of GFR, and since the clearance of mannitol is lower[31,44] than that of inulin ($C_M/C_{IN} = 0.88$) their data for GFR are not suitable to define the normal value. The only data suitable for this purpose are those on C_{IN}.

The most direct approach to characterizing the relation between quantitative values for renal function and increasing age during growth in childhood is accomplished by examining the actual quantitative values for discrete renal functions in subjects at the different ages involved. Actual values obtained for GFR from all available data on C_{IN} in the literature[31-33,43,45,46] are plotted against age in Fig. 3.1. The curve was constructed from mean values obtained for five selected age periods covering birth to 14 years. Individual values for subjects under 6 months of age are not plotted because of space limitations. Even though there is great variation within members of each of the different age groups, a clear pattern of change is apparent. The velocity of change (rate of increase) of GFR is greatest in the first few months of life and thereafter is seen to decrease progressively with each advancing age group even into puberty. The rate of increase does not appear to bear a constant proportionality to age over any two of the time periods chosen. The glomerular filtration rate thus is continuously increasing from birth to maturity but at a gradually decelerating rate.

It is readily apparent that the curve describing the gradual increase in GFR with growth is similar in form to the classical anthropometric serial growth curves constructed from actual measurements of height and weight of children at comparable ages. This form of data presentation shows the cumulative actual achievement of GFR (as is the case with height or weight) at each given age. The speed of the renal growth process is not constant during childhood, as seen by the changing slope of the curve. If one desires to define periods of change in rate of growth, a different presentation is required in which rate of growth can be plotted against age to show changes in growth velocity with advancing age, so-called incremental growth curves.

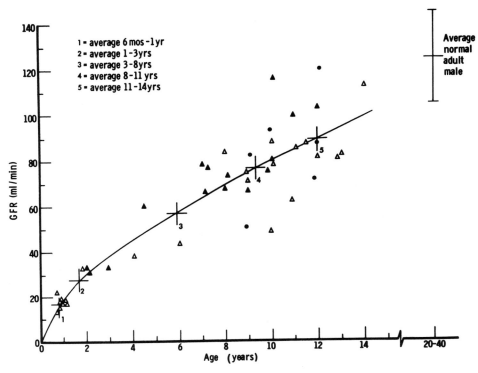

FIGURE 3.1   Mean of actual values for glomerular filtration rate from birth to 14 years of age.   △ = F. K. Friederiszick[35];   ▲ = M. Pérez-Stable[33];   ● = J. B. Richmond et al.[46]

Such incremental growth curves constructed by Tanner, Whitehouse, and Takaishi[47] demonstrate that the highest velocity (rate of increase) for growth of height and weight is seen in the first year of life. The lowest rate is seen after 2 and before 10 to 12 years of age, when a second acceleration in growth rate is seen coincident with the pubertal growth spurt, after which growth stops. The rapid increase in GFR in the first year of life is similar to other changes in body size. The slowing after 2 to 3 years is also similar, but we do not have the necessary data to determine whether an increase in rate of change in renal function again occurs during the period of the accelerated pubertal growth rate. The growth curves for age-related achievement using data for C_{PAH}, Tm_{PAH}, and $Tm_{GLUCOSE}$ would be similar in form to that for GFR. Actual values for these discrete renal functions thus are continuously increasing during the whole period of childhood growth until stable adult values are achieved at maturity (20 years).

There has been surprisingly little interest in using actual values for renal function during growth to define normal values for a given age or to define the changes occurring with increasing age. Early investigators in this field were primarily interested in emphasizing quantitative differences that could be found between renal functions in young infants and adults.[8,32,37] They chose a point of reference that would standardize body size and thereby provide a basis for constant proportionality between body size and renal function during the period of childhood growth and allow comparison with values accepted as normal for adults. West, Smith, and Chasis[37] found that the values for renal function appeared to be constant in children over 3 years of age when surface area was chosen at the common standard of reference; Rubin, Bruck, and Rapoport[32] confirmed their findings.

The latter investigators also compared the curve obtained using actual values for GFR at different ages with that obtained when GFR was related to several different body measurements including body weight, height, surface area, and average kidney weight in grams and average basal metabolic rate; they further compared these different ratios to the values for adults. They found that values for GFR per unit of body weight were lower in newborn infants than in adults, and the values rose above the adult range after 6 months, reaching a peak during the second to third year after which they declined. When GFR was related to height, it increased continuously with age in a pattern similar to that seen when actual values for GFR are plotted against age (see Fig. 3.1). When surface area was used, the values were about 50 percent those of adults at birth. While an occasional value rose to adult levels before 1 year of age, the values were not consistently in the adult range until the second year. Thereafter they remained at a constant level during the rest of childhood.

When kidney weight was used as the reference, the value gradually increased "with maturation being reached between the fourth and fifth month of life."[32] While the data show great variation, Rubin and his associates felt that values throughout childhood were more closely parallel to adult values by this method than any other, even though only crude estimates of kidney weight were available in all subjects. The values for GFR and RPF increase linearly from low values at birth in the young rat[6,24] and in the puppy[25] when related to grams of kidney weight until

they reach constant levels similar to mature animals at about 4 weeks
in the rat and 10 weeks in the puppy. The ratio of GFR per gram
kidney weight is constant during normal growth in rats after 4 to 5
weeks of age.[6]

The achievement of this constant relationship (GFR and RPF

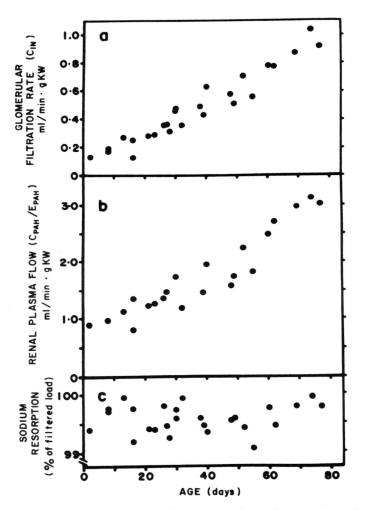

FIGURE 3.2   Relation of glomerular filtration rate (a) and renal plasma flow (b)
to postnatal age. Despite the steadily increasing filtered load of sodium, fractional
sodium resorption for the whole kidney (c) remains constant. (From M. Horster
and H. Valtin.[25])

ml/min/gm kidney wt) has been used by Horster[24,25] to define the time of maturation of renal function in the dog and rat. The data of Horster and Valtin for puppies are shown in Fig. 3.2 and the linearity of the rate of increase is evident. Rubin ultimately chose to define the process of maturation of renal function as being completed when values related to 1.73 m² S.A. became comparable to adult values—by about 3 years of age. This basis for definition of the maturation of renal function in man has now become standard practice.

DISCRETE RENAL FUNCTION RELATED TO A COMMON UNIT OF SURFACE AREA

West, Smith, and Chasis[37] were the first to use surface area as the basis for comparing renal function in infants and children. They felt that relative to aging, renal function in subjects of varying size could best be correlated with the surface area of the average normal adult.

It is now the custom to express all measurements of renal function by correcting the values to 1.73 m² S.A. (the mean value for body surface area of the "normal" adult male). The studies of Barnett[8] and subsequently many others[32–35,43,45,46,48] have demonstrated that the mean values for GFR (C_{IN}), RPF (C_{PAH}), and tubular mass (Tm_{PAH} and $Tm_{GLUCOSE}$) are quite low in young infants when compared to values of adults on this basis. All suitable data from the literature reporting values for these various renal functions in normal newborn infants, premature infants, and children—corrected to 1.73 m² S.A.—are presented in Table 3.3.

When these values are expressed as percentages of the normal adult values, it is apparent that values for GFR are not so low even in the youngest infants as those for RPF (C_{PAH}) and tubular mass (Tm_{PAH}). As stated earlier, the value of C_{PAH} is less than the actual value of minimal effective RPF until after 6 months of age, and values for effective RPF obtained from C_{PAH} in the infant under 3 months of age need to be revised upward by at least 30 percent. The value of RPF (C_{PAH}) is, however, still lower in infants 6 months to 1 year (54 percent of normal) than GFR (62 percent) or Tm_{PAH} (64 percent). After 1 year all three values continue to increase proportionally to reach levels generally similar to those for adults in children older than 3 years of age, then appear to stabilize at this level.

This observation has led to the conclusion that values in subjects over

TABLE 3.3   Comparison of renal function in infants and children with that in adults. All values are corrected to 1.73 m² S.A.

Age[a]	Number of cases	GFR (C_{IN}) ml/min	% of adult	C_{PAH} ml/min	% of adult	Tm_{PAH} mg/min	% of adult	$Tm_{GLUCOSE}$ mg/min	% of adult	Reference no.
Newborn	43	26 ± 1.7	21	88 ± 4.2	13					43
3 days old	26	36 ± 3.9	30	134 ± 14.3	24					43
1–2 weeks	6	54 ± 8.0	44							45
P: 1–2 weeks	6	50 ± 10.0	40	154 ± 34	24	13 ± 6	17	70.6 ± 19.6	19	31, 34, 49
P: 1–2 months	9					16.1 ± 5.2	20	105.3 ± 27.2	28	31, 34, 49
2–4 months	9	56 ± 10.0	44	234 ± 50	36					35
P: 2–5 months	6	68 ± 21.0	55	222 ± 60	34	24 ± 15	30	170 ± 5[c]	45	31, 34, 49
6 months–1 year	6	77 ± 14.0	62	352 ± 73	54	51 ± 20 M[b]	64			32, 35
1–3 years	6	96 ± 22.0	77	537 ± 122	80	66 ± 19 M	82			32, 33, 35
3–8 years	8	131 ± 26	105	659 ± 115	101	65 ± 24 M	81			32, 33, 35
8–14 years	13	120 ± 20	96	631 ± 98	96	77 ± 20 M	96			46
20–40 years										
Male		125 ± 19	100	655 ± 98	100	80 ± 12	100	375 ± 56	100	9
Female		110 ± 17	100	570 ± 86	100	77 ± 11	100	303 ± 45	100	9

[a] P = prematurely born.
[b] M = mannitol used to measure GFR.
[c] Two observations.

3 years of age are identical to those in adults[32] when comparison is related to a unit of surface area. Such a conclusion seems reasonable with respect to values for GFR (C_{IN}) and RPF (C_{PAH}), but the number of observations on Tm_{PAH} and $Tm_{GLUCOSE}$ in subjects over 6 months of age is quite limited. The only available data for values for Tm_{PAH} in children older than 5 months are those of Rubin, Bruck, and Rapoport.[32] Since these authors used mannitol to measure GFR, their values for Tm_{PAH} are subject to error and the true mean value for Tm_{PAH} is probably lower than their mean value. Galán and his colleagues[49] found a higher value for $Tm_{GLUCOSE}$ (583 mg/min $\pm$ 130 per 1.73 m² S.A.) in six normal children 2 to 12 years of age than that reported in adults (375 mg/min $\pm$ 15 percent for males). The available data are too limited to define normal values for Tm_{PAH} and $Tm_{GLUCOSE}$ in older children.

I have not followed the usual practice when describing normal values for discrete renal functions in children, which is to give a single value for all children older than 2 years of age up to 12 to 14 years of age.[50] The data in Table 3.3 have been divided into age groups similar to those used to provide mean values for Fig. 3.1 in order to facilitate broader age-related comparison. This exercise is obviously precluded when data from 2 to 14 years are pooled. The differences apparent in mean values for GFR, RPF, and Tm_{PAH} for subjects 1 to 3, 3 to 8, and 8 to 14 years could represent meaningful variations—but they could as easily be physiologically nonsignificant variations, since the number of observations is small and the variation between individuals large relative to the mean.

The practice of pooling data over this large time span of childhood growth (2 to 14 years) may be justifiable statistically if one seeks only to define the most reliable mean value with the limited data, but it hides our ignorance about the constancy of values for renal function when related to standard surface area throughout such a long span of active growth. Separation of children between 2 and 14 years of age into subgroups may be considered a labor of love, but it calls attention to the need to examine changes in renal function during childhood growth in a serial manner before we jump to the conclusion that no significant changes occur relative to aging after 2 to 3 years of age.

The comparison with standards for normal adult values poses a special problem when dealing with infants, since actual values are less than 50 percent of adult values at birth and are increasing continuously from birth up to 2 to 3 years of age when they equal adult values. Mean values for the normal GFR related to surface area in infants under 2 years can be obtained when they are standardized for age rather than expressed as percent subnormal by adult standards. Winberg[51] has constructed a curve that gives mean values for normal GFR in young infants using the endogenous C_{CR}, which he demonstrated correlates well with values obtained by C_{IN}. A curve constructed from his data to relate actual value per 1.73 m² S.A. to age in infancy is shown in Fig. 3.3. This allows the physician to judge whether the actual value (attainment) related to surface area in an infant below 2 years of age falls within the normal range observed in subjects of comparable age.

The 24-hour true endogenous creatinine clearance is a useful method for estimation of GFR in healthy children, but it is often higher than C_{IN} in children with renal disease because of tubular secretion of creatinine.[52] Another source of error arises from the contribution of serum noncreatinine chromogens to the Jaffe reaction when protein-free filtrates

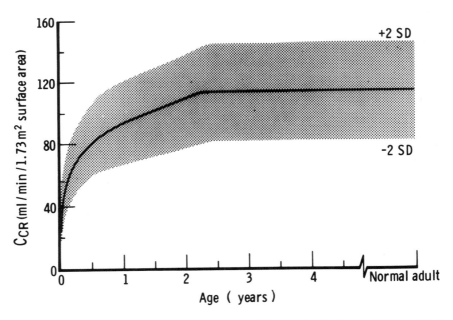

FIGURE 3.3   Changes in normal value for GFR standardized to ml/1.73 m² S.A. from birth into later childhood. The GFR is measured by the endogenous creatinine clearance (C_{CR}) corrected to 1.73 m² S.A. The solid line depicts the mean value and the shaded area includes ±2 standard deviations. Data are adapted from J. Winberg.[51]

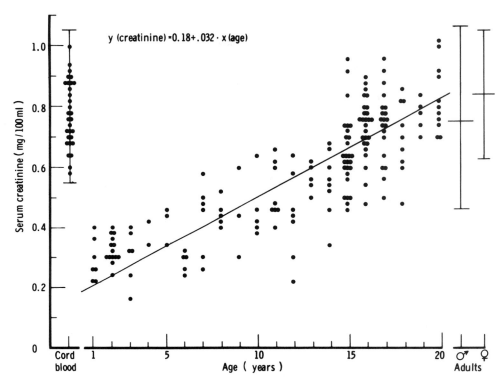

FIGURE 3.4 Serum creatinine in relation to age. (From B. Kuhlbäck et al.[54])

are used; this error is greatest when one is dealing with low true serum creatinine levels.[53] The level of true serum creatinine is continuously rising from the low levels in infancy to reach adult levels at about 20 years.[54] The normal serum creatinine level thus varies with age during childhood (see Fig. 3.4). The error arising from the measurement of serum creatinine by direct reading without prior elution of creatinine (the commonly used method in clinical chemistry laboratories) is insignificant when creatinine is at or above normal adult levels,[55] but could be significant with the low serum creatinine levels found in infants.

When true endogenous creatinine clearances were measured by the method of Hare employing elution of creatinine by Lloyd's reagent in twenty-two normal infants, children, and adults,[55] the average ratio of C_{CR}/C_{IN} was 1.03. The errors associated with the use of the endogenous C_{CR} as a measure of GFR have led some observers to consider it an unreliable measure.[56] As stated above, however, if care is taken to eliminate bedside collection errors and 24-hour collections are employed with measurement of true serum creatinine by the elution method of Hare, the C_{CR} is a useful and reliable estimate of GFR in normal subjects.[10,51,55]

EXPLANATION OF LOW VALUES FOR TUBULAR TRANSPORT CAPACITY IN INFANTS

The values for maximal tubular transport activity (Tm_{PAH} and $Tm_{GLUCOSE}$) are lower in infants when compared with adults than the values for GFR and RPF. This has been attributed to underdevelopment of renal tubular cellular organization and enzyme activity. The development of "adult values" for maximal tubular transport capacity requires cellular maturation of individual cells comprising the tubules as well as growth in size to allow immature nephrons to elongate and hypertrophy to "catch up" to the continuously increasing glomerular volume delivered during early postnatal growth. There is direct evidence from in vitro studies of cellular underdevelopment (immaturity).

The capacity of the renal cortex to accumulate the organic acid PAH and the organic base tetraethylammonium has been shown to be lower in renal cortical slices in vitro in tissues from fetal and newborn rabbits, puppies, and piglets than from adults.[57,58] Rennick, Hamilton, and Evans[58] found that the two systems in puppies matured independently postnatally but both reached adult levels at about 9 weeks of age. Of equal interest is their demonstration that the transport activity of tissues from the superficial layer of the cortex was less than that of cortical tissues from deeper layers of the young kidney of the rabbit. They correlated these findings with histologic evidence that the superficial nephrons were morphologically less well developed than those in the deeper layers at birth.

Baxter and Yoffey[59] have also provided evidence that tubular transport activity in the immature superficial proximal tubules is less well developed in the newborn rat than in the more mature ones in the deeper cortex (see Chapter 1). The interesting report of Priestly and Malt[60] on cellular nucleic acid synthesis in the developing rat kidney indicates that significant changes also occur in intracellular membrane organization in the immediate postnatal period. These findings indicate some of the steps involved in cellular maturation leading to enhanced renal tubular transport capacity; they will be discussed further in Chapter 5.

PROBLEMS ENCOUNTERED IN RELATING RENAL FUNCTION TO BODY SIZE

The definition of renal functional maturation on the basis of disappearance of significant differences between values for renal function in children and adults when both are related to a common unit of surface area is empiric and open to question. It also implies that the intrarenal functional and autoregulatory circulatory adjustments controlling overall glomerular tubular balance during the rest of childhood growth (after 2 to 3 years of age) are identical to those that exist after growth ceases with sexual maturity. The biochemical and physiologic validity of these assumptions has yet to be established.

A further problem concerns the variation of normal values for adults with age and sex. Values for all renal functions average about 10 percent less in the female than in the male,[61] and Davies and Shock have reported[62] that values for GFR, RPF, and maximal tubular transport capacity ($Tm_{DIODRAST}$) fall progressively after 40 years of age, as shown in Figs. 3.5 and 3.6. The gradual decrease in values for GFR and RPF involves a slightly greater decrease in the latter than the former, and the filtration fraction consequently rises slightly with advancing age. The adult value must therefore be defined by sex and age.

There are theoretical and physiologic limitations inherent in the use of surface area as the standard for any such comparison of organ function with variable physical parameters. The selection of any basis that involves a derived ratio (GFR/S.A.) introduces possibilities for misinterpretation because of spurious hidden correlation, as Tanner has convincingly pointed out.[63] This procedure is also unsuitable for the detection of changes in the rate of maturation (velocity increase) in two groups of comparable age. If one desires to determine by group comparison what effect a particular stimulus (such as starvation or a high-protein diet) may have in altering the rate of increase in a specific aspect of renal function changing normally during a particular period of growth, correction to surface area standards could obscure any changes present between groups.

The major attraction of this practice is that it allows comparison to be made between values for adults and for infants since both are expressed in terms of a common unit of surface area. Since this practice is presently used as the basis for most interpretations of changes in renal function during growth, as well as for the definition of the time of

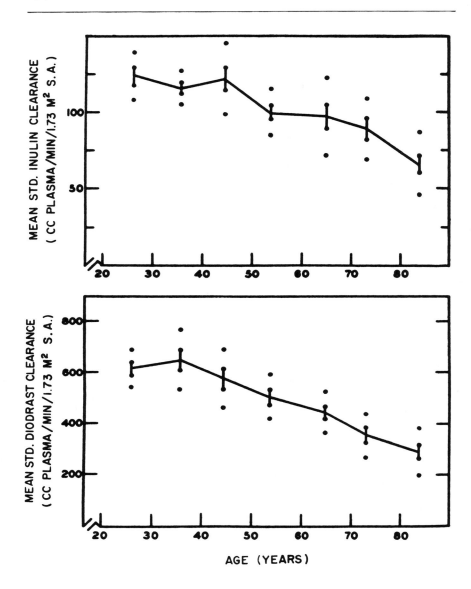

FIGURE 3.5 Average change in standard inulin clearance or glomerular filtration rate with age, and average change in standard diodrast clearance or effective renal plasma flow with age. The vertical lines represent ±1 standard deviation of the mean; the circles represent ±1 standard deviation of the distribution. (From D. F. Davies and N. W. Shock.[62])

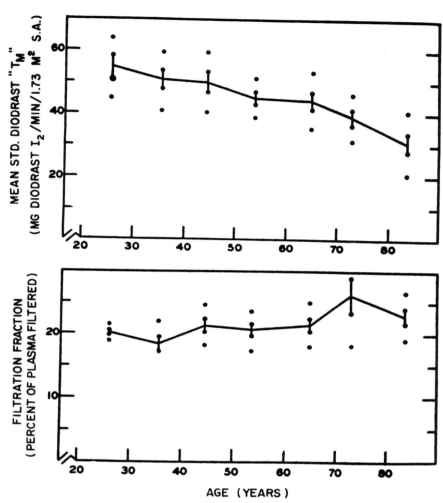

FIGURE 3.6 Average change in standard diodrast Tm with age, and average change in filtration fraction with age. The vertical lines represent ±1 standard deviation of the mean; the circles represent ±1 standard deviation of the distribution. (From D. F. Davies and N. W. Shock.[62])

maturation of renal function, some discussion of the pitfalls and limitations inherent in its use seems appropriate at this time.

The fact that no difference can be shown to exist in values for renal function with the use of surface area standardization between children and adults, when it is obvious that differences do exist in the velocity of growth, volume of total body water, extracellular fluid, and the like, serves to emphasize how this practice hides their interrelations with renal function during growth. The selection of a basis for comparison that eliminates variation when it is not only known to exist but also to bear some physiologic relationship to the function in question (that is, GFR and extracellular fluid volume) may be justified only if useful information not otherwise available is gained thereby.

This approach may also obscure the opportunities for recognition of direct relationships present but changing during the period of growth. The possibility that there are changing but nonetheless direct relationships between actual values of renal function and the volume of body fluids during growth is of particular interest. It may be more appropriate to relate renal function to total body water or extracellular fluid volume than to surface area. It is now generally recognized that renal function is intimately involved in the regulation of normal body fluid volume and composition. It can readily be shown that induced alterations in the volume of body fluid compartments, especially the vascular compartment and extracellular fluid volume, can have direct effects on quantitative values for GFR and RPF and on renal tubular resorption of salt and water in mature subjects. Acute changes in these extrarenal factors influence renal function in young subjects as well, as studies have demonstrated.[64]

McCance and Widdowson[65] have questioned the validity of choosing surface area as the optimal basis for assessment of changes in renal function during growth. While granting the existence of proportionality between kidney function and metabolic rate and surface area during growth and aging, they proposed that more physiologic comparative evaluations of renal functions between subjects of different ages would be obtained if the parameter chosen had a more direct functional association with the regulatory responsibility of the function being tested.

Tubular transport of sodium and water and GFR are largely responsible for renal regulation of the volume of body water. The volume of total body water in the infant after 6 months of age constitutes approximately 60 percent of the body weight, as is the case in the adult male. Accordingly, McCance and Widdowson proposed that GFR be related for purposes of comparison to the volume of body water found in the average normal adult (42 liters). If 42 liters of body water is chosen as the standard and values in small subjects are expressed in this way, as they suggest, the type of curve found with aging is different than when actual values are used or when corrected to 1.73 m² S.A., as is evident from Fig. 3.7.

The values for GFR are lowest at birth by all methods. Every curve rises rapidly during the first 6 months of life. The curve based on 42 liters of body water rises to a peak at 5 to 6 years, reaching levels almost twice those found in adults. It then remains elevated relative to adult values throughout childhood growth, finally falling to reach adult values in late adolescence. When 1.73 m² S.A. is chosen as the basis of comparison, the form of the curve is similar to that seen when actual values are plotted against age, but the adult value is achieved at an earlier

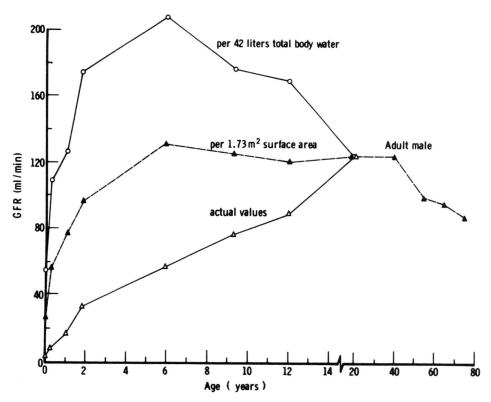

FIGURE 3.7   Changes in mean value for GFR with age (△), when related to 1.73 m² S.A. (▲) and when related to 42 liters of body water (○). Points used to construct curve represent mean values for birth, 2 to 4 months, ½ to 1 year, 1 to 3 years, 3 to 8 years, 8 to 11 years, and 11 to 14 years. Values for adult male are taken from D. F. Davies and N. W. Shock.[62]

age—3 years. In the latter two instances, however, the values virtually never exceed those found in adults. The significance of these differences may be appreciated more fully if we consider the data now available describing the changes occurring in the size of body fluid compartments during growth.

Friis-Hansen[66] has shown that the volume of total body water changes in a nonlinear manner during growth, whether related to age or units of surface area or body weight, when comparisons include infants and adults. The lack of constant proportionality is the result of concomitant changes occurring in lean body mass and in the volume of intracellular and extracellular fluid compartments during growth and aging. Data describing these relations with aging are shown in Table 3.4. When the volume of total body water is expressed as a percentage of body weight, it is greatest at birth (77 percent), decreases to 62 percent by 6 months of age, but thereafter remains relatively constant into adolescence. A constant relationship thus can be seen to exist between the two after 6 months of age, and it persists until sex differences appear at puberty. The relationship then continues to be linear in the male but ceases to be so in the female because of the deposition of fat which lowers the percentage of body weight represented by water.[67]

When the actual values for total body water volume are related to surface area, the volume is now lowest at birth, being about 22 liters/1.73 m² S.A. and it increases continuously though slowly during all of childhood. The sex differences again become apparent at puberty and the

TABLE 3.4   Changes in volume of total body water and extracellular space with growth when related to surface area and as a function of body weight (from B. Friis-Hansen[66] and I. S. Edelman et al.[67])

Age	Total body water		Extracellular space	
	1/1.73 m² S.A.	% body wt	1/1.73 m² S.A.	% body wt
0–11 days	21.8	77	11.8	42
11–120 days	21.3	73	10.0	34
½–2 years	23.7	62	10.0	27
2–7 years	25.4	63	10.0	25
10–15 years (male)	33.2	59	12.0	20
12–15 years (female)	30.5	56	12.0	20
17–34 years (male)	40.5	61	18.0	18
20–31 years (female)	31.2	51	14.2	19

value at maturity in males (40.5 1/1.73 m² S.A.) is considerably above that found in females at maturity (31.2 1/1.73 m² S.A.). Both values decline slowly thereafter with aging.

The relation between total body water volume and body weight thus differs from that between the former and surface area during growth and in the two sexes after sexual maturation. The proportion of body weight represented by total body water is continuously decreasing from the time of birth on into adulthood, whereas when total body water volume is related to a common unit of surface area it increases from birth up to sexual maturity and then decreases in old age.[67] The shape of a curve describing the relationship of total body water in 1/1.73 m² S.A. would be similar to that seen when GFR/1.73 m² S.A. is related to age as in Fig. 3.7. As has already been pointed out, when GFR is related to a common unit of surface area and plotted against age from birth to maturity, it rises up to 2 to 3 years of age, remains constant up to 40 years of age, and then falls.

The curve obtained by relating GFR to a common unit of body water and plotting this against age differs in its growth pattern, however, from that obtained when surface area is chosen as the standard of reference. When GFR is related to total body water volume during growth and aging, it rises to a maximal value at 5 to 6 years and thereafter progressively declines in the manner of an aging process! This is clearly a different growth and aging pattern for GFR from that observed using the conventional practice of relating GFR to surface area. These differences in curves describing growth patterns with aging are pointed out to emphasize the unavoidable difficulties faced when renal function in infants and adults is compared by relating it to any arbitrary standard of reference that is not itself proportional or constant during aging in the two populations under study.

It is evident from Table 3.4 that no constant proportionality exists between body weight and total body water or extracellular volume during any prolonged period of growth. When the values for extracellular fluid volume are related to surface area, however, they do remain constant (10 1/1.73 m² S.A.) after the first 6 months of life up to the adolescent period (10 to 15 years), when further increases occur ending in higher values for mature males (18 1/1.73 m² S.A.) than for females (14.2 1/1.73 m² S.A.). The long period during which there is a constant relation between extracellular volume and surface area (2 to 10 years of age) coincides with and might account for the constancy observed when values for GFR or RPF are related to a common unit of surface area in the same age of childhood, as pointed out by Friis-Hansen.[66]

A more meaningful basis for the comparative study of renal function during childhood growth and aging might be to correlate GFR with extracellular fluid volume. The absence of simple methods for accurate measurement of this compartment precludes such a practice. The observation that GFR appears to achieve levels comparable to those of adults at 2 to 3 years of age when related to surface area, and to stay at these levels into maturity, remains valid; however, it may be a spurious correlation and its physiologic and developmental significance remains to be established.

GLOMERULOTUBULAR INTERRELATIONS DURING GROWTH

Anatomic Correlates of Glomerulotubular Balance

The increase in size and function of the kidney during growth is associated with changes in physical dimensions of the individual nephrons. The striking heterogeneity of nephrons and localization of small nephrons to the outer cortex that characterizes the newborn kidney has largely disappeared by 6 months to 1 year. The growth of nephrons involves all of their parts. There is a progressive increase in size and diameter of the glomerulus with adult lobulation developing in the second to third year of life. Since the volume of a sphere increases with the cube of the radius, the adult glomerulus with a mean diameter of 0.283 mm could have a volume about fifteen times greater than the infant glomerulus with a mean diameter of 0.116 mm.

The length of proximal tubules has been measured by Fetterman[22] and by Darmady and his associates[68] during growth and the average length has been related to age. The length of the proximal tubule does not approach that of the adult until late adolescence. Darmady's finding of unusually short proximal tubules (about one-half the expected length) in kidneys of children with nephrogenic diabetes insipidus and cystinosis suggests that abnormal anatomic development may be involved in these renal diseases. The average length of the proximal tubule apparently is not stationary once sexual maturation has occurred, since Darmady has found[69] that there is a progressive slow decrease in average length of proximal tubules in adult kidneys after 40 to 50 years of age—sufficient to amount to a decrease in mean length of about one-third by 80 years of age, as shown in Table 3.5.

There is also a decrease in mean glomerular surface area with aging. This is of special interest in view of the previously cited data of Davies and Shock[62] showing that there is a progressive decline in renal function associated with aging.

The functional correlates that can be derived from the morphologic evidence of "immaturity" have been strikingly developed by Fetterman and his colleagues[22] in their application of Oliver's concept of *structural-functional equivalence* in the nephron.[70] By this concept the quantitative relations of glomerular and tubular structural dimensions are compared with Smith's analysis by clearances of the functional activity of glomerulo-tubular balance in the handling of glucose by the nephrons. Smith's ratios,[71] the expression of this functional balance, were found by Oliver to be reproducible from the measurements of the two concerned structural elements, glomerulus and proximal convolution, where the functional activities of filtration and resorption were occurring. Their substitution in Smith's formulas thus afforded the means for constructing the "titration curve" with its characteristic splay from the morphologic data. A similar result was obtained by Bradley and his associates[29] in their examination of the nephron of the dog.

Fetterman and his co-workers[22] made measurements needed to derive quantitative estimates of mean glomerular surface area (SGA) and mean volume of the proximal convolutions (the product of proximal tubular diameter and length and abbreviated as PV) and then estimated the

TABLE 3.5 Changes in dimensions of nephrons with growth and aging in man (from E. M. Darmady, *Journal of Pathology*, in press)

No. of cases	Age range (yrs)	Proximal length (mm)	Proximal volume (mm³)	Glomerular surface area (mm²)	Mean R value
13	Term–9	7.12	0.022	0.083	9.91
12	10–19	14.91	0.050	0.201	6.70
21	20–39	19.36	0.076	0.254	3.17
19	40–59	18.12	0.073	0.262	3.52
12	60–69	17.38	0.067	0.222	3.30
13	70–79	16.17	0.061	0.179	2.97
15	80–101	12.50	0.052	0.155	3.34

glomerulotubular balance (GSA/PV) based on morphologic data during
growth from birth to maturity. They studied nephrons in the outer,
middle, and inner cortex of the kidney in twenty-two normal subjects
from birth to 18 years of age.

The value of the ratio of GSA/PV for the individual nephrons is
termed r; the mean value for r of all nephrons in the kidney is designated
R. Oliver and MacDowell[70] found this to be the best anatomic expression
for quantitative assessment of glomerulotubular balance. The term R
relates proximal tubular volume (PV) to glomerular activity (GSA)
on the basis of anatomic estimates in terms similar to those used by
Smith.[71] Smith defined overall functional glomerulotubular balance by
using the rate of filtration of glucose to measure glomerular load and
relate it to functional capacity for tubular resorption (of glucose)[29] as
measured by $Tm_{GLUCOSE}$.

Nephrons with large tubular resorptive capacity relative to glomerular
volume have a low value for r and those with small resorptive capacity
relative to glomerular volume have a high ratio for r. The mean value
of R for the composite adult kidney found by Oliver and MacDowell
was 3.22 with a variation in r values of 1.86 to 6.58. In the full-term
infant the value of R found by the Fetterman group was quite high,
27.9 (see Table 3.6). This indicates that there is proportionally greater
overall glomerular activity relative to tubular function in the newborn
kidney than that found in the adult. The high mean value for R decreases
rapidly to 7.8 by 6 months (Table 3.6) and thereafter falls more slowly.
It decreases gradually throughout the rest of childhood, but Fetterman
found that it does not equal the adult value of 3.17 even at 18 years
of age.

Essentially identical values for GSA/PV or R in children have been
obtained by Darmady using similar techniques. The value of R remained
above that found in adults in subjects up to 19 years of age (Table
3.5). The lowest values of R found by Darmady in subjects less than
20 years of age were 3.96 and 3.84 in the kidney of a 17- and an 18-year-
old male respectively.[69]

The distribution of small and large nephrons in a specific area of
the cortex was also measured by examination of the range of values
for r. It was apparent that their distribution differed in the newborn
kidney from that of the adult. The majority of r values for individual
nephrons fell to the left of the mean value of R for the composite kidney
in the newborn. Such "skewing" to the left indicates that in the newborn

TABLE 3.6 Interrelations among renal functions during growth. The GFR is measured by C_{IN} unless otherwise noted.

Age[a]	Number of cases	GFR/C_{PAH}	GFR/Tm_{PAH}	GFR/$Tm_{GLUCOSE}$	C_{PAH}/Tm_{PAH}	R (GSA/PV)[b] Mean	Range	Reference no.
Newborn	34	0.31 ± 0.03				27.9	4.7–97.5	43
P: 3–13 days	8	0.34 ± 0.06	3.8 ± 1.4		11.2 ± 3.8			31
P: 7–30 days	9			0.51 ± 0.05				34, 49
P: 1–2 months	9	0.33 ± 0.06	4.4 ± 1.7		10.9 ± 3.4			31, 34
P: 1–2 months	8			0.47 ± 0.04				34, 49
P: 3–5 months	2			0.35 ± 0.04				34
P: 2–5 months	6	0.31 ± 0.06	3.3 ± 1.2		9.2 ± 3.5	10.1	3.6–19.5	31, 34
½–1 year	6	0.22 ± 0.06	1.5(M)[c] ± 1.5		6.9(M)[c] ± 3.5	7.8	3.2–20.1	32, 35
1–3 years	6	0.18 ± 0.05	1.5(M) ± 1.2		8.1(M) ± 4.3	5.9	2.5–22.8	32, 35
3–8 years	8	0.20 ± 0.05	2.0(M) ± 0.5		10.1(M) ± 1.6	6.6	3.1–18.6	32, 35
8–14 years	13	0.19 ± 0.04	1.6(M) ± 0.7		8.2(M) ± 2.3	5.6	2.1–13.8	32, 35
2–12 years	6			0.27 ± 0.08				50
Adults								
Male		0.19 ± 0.03	1.6 ± 0.4	0.33 ± 0.05	8.2 ± 2.0	3.17	1.9–6.6	9
Female		0.19 ± 0.03	1.5 ± 0.4	0.36 ± 0.05	7.4 ± 2.0	3.17	1.9–6.6	9

[a] P = prematurely born.
[b] R = GSA/PV = ratio of glomerular surface area to proximal tubular volume from data of G. H. Fetterman et al.[22]
[c] M = mannitol used to measure GFR.

kidney the majority of the nephrons have lower glomerular activity (r/R is less than 1.0) than the mean value for the composite kidney (R). This is a reflection of the large number of immature nephrons with small glomeruli that are found in the outer cortex.

The greater spread in range of values for r/R is further evidence that wide diversity in dimensional glomerulotubular relationships is a characteristic of the nephrons of the newborn kidney. Even though the range of variation in dimensions of individual nephrons (heterogeneity) was great in the newborn, there appeared to be allometry (matching to preserve parity of glomerulotubular balance) since the shortest proximal tubules generally had the smallest glomeruli and vice versa. The speed with which allometric growth corrects heterogeneity is evident from the histogram of the 2-year-old, which closely resembles that of the adult. This similarity is depicted in Fig. 3.8. The disappearance of heterogeneity occurs even earlier than 2 years of age, since Fetterman and his co-workers comment: "By 3½ months, however, the histogram of nephrons in any kidney shows the same general configuration as that of the adult, expressive of a similar heterogeneity."[22] These investigators provided anatomic evidence that this major sign of immaturity has largely disappeared by 6 months of age.

There has been some criticism voiced concerning the reliability of measurements of isolated nephrons.[72,73] Elias and Hennig[73] found lower values for glomerular diameters than those of Fetterman and Darmady; however, they did not use microdissection but rather made measurements from cut sections of fixed tissues. The actual value of R will differ depending on the method employed, but it seems improbable that the differences found between values of R in kidneys of children by Fetterman and his associates[22] and Darmady[69] and those of adults by Oliver and MacDowell[70] can be ascribed to methodologic error alone. Fetterman comments as follows: "We are convinced of the reliability of such measurements in the hands of experienced, capable dissectors. As in all quantitative procedures proper control is required and the final test of validity is reproducibility: the results in our laboratory and those of Oliver [70] and Darmady [69] are practically interchangeable." Fetterman's R value in adult kidneys is similar[74] to that reported by Oliver.

Morphometric analysis of intracortical distribution of number and volume of glomeruli during postnatal maturation in the dog by Horster, Kemler, and Valtin[75] revealed a systematic pattern in the dog suggestive of two populations of glomeruli in the mature animal. In studies initiated

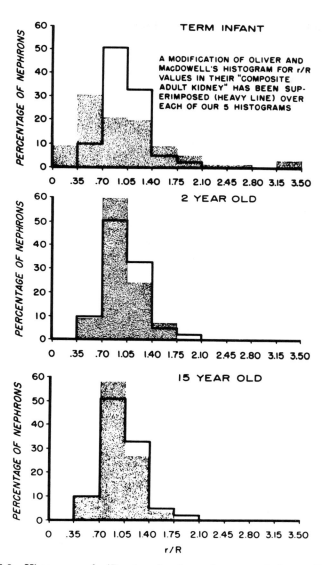

FIGURE 3.8 Histograms of r/R values for the nephron population studied in each of three subjects beginning with the term infant. The resemblance of the histograms in the 2- and 15-year-old to the superimposed histogram of comparable values from the composite adult kidney is striking.

after completion of postnatal nephronogenesis (3 weeks after birth in the normal dog), there was no change by 77 days after birth in number or in qualitative differences in mean glomerular volume at different cortical levels, except for those in the subcapsular level which were smallest at 23 days but increased to levels similar to the other cortical glomeruli by 74 days. The juxtamedullary glomeruli were consistently larger than the cortical glomeruli. The pattern of nephron maturation was related to age and cortical location. Postnatal functional maturation during the period of study was accompanied by an increase of about 33 percent in glomerular volume. Tubular growth was preponderant over glomerular growth in early postnatal maturation, as is the case in the human.

The explanation proposed by Fetterman and his co-workers[22] for the higher value of R in children as compared with adults was that it reflected the smaller individual proximal tubular volume in relation to glomerular surface. The higher R value was the result of a smaller proximal tubular diameter, since it was still present when nephrons from children were measured that were matched according to proximal tubular length for those obtained in the adult. If the constancy of the value of R can be accepted as anatomic evidence of glomerular tubular balance, it would appear that it becomes relatively stable after 6 months of age decreasing only slowly thereafter into adolescence and that it differs during childhood growth from that found in the mature 35-year-old adult.

Fetterman concluded that "the last step in maturation of an individual convolution is an increase in tubular volume, caused not by further lengthening of the tubule, but rather by an increase in its diameter. An accompaniment of this final increase in volume in any one nephron is a decrease in gs/pv ratio (r)." The possibility that this finding has physiologic significance and is not the result of a methodologic effect unique to microdissection deserves consideration. If it has a physiologic correlate, it would be that glomerulotubular balance during the period of active growth in childhood may be maintained by a different interplay of the regulatory forces responsible after body growth has ceased.

Functional Relation between GFR, RPF, and Total Tubular Mass (Tm_{PAH} and $Tm_{GLUCOSE}$)

The ratio of GFR and RPF to functional tubular mass as measured by Tm_{PAH} and $Tm_{GLUCOSE}$ can be examined during growth to determine what the relationships are and to reveal any pattern of change. Changes in these ratios during early growth will reflect only composite function of all nephrons, but it could reveal something about the nature of the qualitative intrarenal functional adjustments that exist in the maturing kidney while nephron size is changing with growth.

The overall glomerulotubular balance can be evaluated by calculating the ratio of filtration rate per unit of functioning tubular mass (C_{IN}/Tm_{PAH} and C_{IN}/$Tm_{GLUCOSE}$). The blood flow per unit of tubular function can be estimated by calculating the ratio of blood flow (C_{PAH}) per unit of functioning tubular mass measured as either C_{PAH}/Tm_{PAH} or C_{PAH}/$Tm_{GLUCOSE}$. The filtration fraction is estimated by C_{IN}/C_{PAH}.

The values for these ratios at different ages in childhood and in adults are shown in Table 3.6. The values for C_{PAH}/Tm_{PAH} in infants less than 6 months of age are high, but they do not have the same validity as they do after 6 months of age for the reasons mentioned above. Furthermore, the value for filtration fraction (GFR/C_{PAH}) in infants under 6 months is not a valid estimate because C_{PAH} does not accurately measure effective renal plasma flow. It is a valid estimate of RPF after that time. The slight elevation of the value to 0.22 seen between 6 months and 1 year is probably not significant since after 1 year of age the mean value appears to be identical to that found in adults (0.18). The data indicate that filtration fraction is similar to that of adults in infants above 1 year of age and may be similar after 6 months of age.

The blood supply per unit of tubular mass (C_{PAH}/Tm_{PAH}) is higher in young infants than in adults but overlaps after 6 months of age. These findings must be interpreted with some caution because the Tm_{PAH} data in subjects over 6 months of age are based on measurements involving the use of mannitol[32] to measure GFR. The high values suggest that the blood supply per unit of tubular mass in infants is certainly not lower than that found in the adult kidney and that there may be hyperemia during his period of rapid growth. It would be most pronounced in early infancy, since C_{PAH} underestimates the effective RPF and the actual RPF/Tm_{PAH} value would be even higher than that derived from C_{PAH}/Tm_{PAH}.

The ratio of filtration rate per unit of functioning tubular mass in infants less than 6 months old is high whether measured by GFR/Tm_{PAH} or GFR/$Tm_{GLUCOSE}$ compared with values in older children and adults. This is in agreement with the morphologic evidence that glomerular activity is greater than tubular activity. The ratio measured by GFR/Tm_{PAH} is similar to that of adults after 6 months of age and throughout the remaining period of childhood studied. There is no functional evidence from the data now available to suggest that glomerular preponderance persists after 6 months of age, but variations in individual nephrons in different cortical levels could be present that are not apparent from the data at hand.

Although the data for $C_{IN}/Tm_{GLUCOSE}$ are limited to prematurely born infants, they are of special interest with respect to the time required to accommodate tubular activity to glomerular load in the postnatal period. The value in the youngest (premature) infants—in other words, the smallest—is higher (0.51 to 0.47) than in adults (0.33), but it has fallen to the adult range in the two oldest prematures studied ($3\frac{1}{3}$ and $4\frac{1}{2}$ months of age). The data on GFR/Tm_{PAH} suggest that the value stabilizes at the adult range by 6 months and remains at this level throughout childhood.

The only data in older children on $GFR/Tm_{GLUCOSE}$ are those of Galán and his colleagues,[49] who found a wide range and a lower mean value for $GFR/Tm_{GLUCOSE}$ than for adults (Table 3.6). Since the range of individual variation in values for $GFR/Tm_{GLUCOSE}$ is considerably less (S.D. $\pm$ 10 percent) than that found for GFR/Tm_{PAH} (S.D. $\pm$ 38 percent), the former appears to provide the more precise index for evaluating change in glomerulotubular balance during growth.

It is of interest that Potter and his associates[6] found that the value for $GFR/Tm_{GLUCOSE}$ was slightly lower in 5- to 7-week-old 175-gm rats than in 350-gm rats, even though the ratio of GFR/gm kidney weight was constant after 4 to 5 weeks of age. This would be compatible with a slight continuing preponderance of GFR relative to $Tm_{GLUCOSE}$ in the young actively growing rat when compared to that found in the mature but still slowly growing 350-gm rats. The results suggest that studies of this type during growth should employ both measurements (Tm_{PAH} and $Tm_{GLUCOSE}$), since tubular secretory and resorptive activity may not always increase in parallel during the period of growth.

The overlap of mean values for GFR/Tm_{PAH} in infants over 6 months of age and older children with those of adults suggests that the functional consequences of the anatomic imbalance between glomerular and tubular function present at birth have largely been corrected by 6 months of age. This seems to be at variance with the anatomic data of Fetterman and his co-workers[22] that show a persistently high value of R (GSA/PV) relative to that of adults throughout the period of childhood growth.

When nephrons grow in size, we know they must also change in function. There is very active interest now in studying the mechanisms responsible for maintaining glomerular tubular balance in the nephrons of the mature subject's kidney. One aspect of these studies is directed toward defining the functional changes associated with renal growth stimulated by a number of situations such as chronic renal failure,[76] unilateral ureteral obstruction,[77,78] or uninephrectomy,[79] that result in compensatory renal hypertrophy. There is need to examine these same functional interrelationships more critically by new studies during the period of postnatal maturation in young growing subjects.

Most of the models used to observe how nephrons change in function when they grow involve study of the growth response stimulated by the removal of renal tissue in the mature animal. When the kidney enlarges by compensatory hypertrophy of the remaining nephrons, there is an increase in glomerular filtration which exceeds the increase in kidney size and weight.[80] The adaptation of the renal tubules to the increased absorptive work resulting from additional fluid filtered is the subject of much present study which is discussed more fully in Chapter 5; for now it suffices to point out that the growing (and maturing) kidney of the young subject is also an example of renal growth hypertrophy, even though it is primary rather than compensatory hypertrophy.

Information derived from the application of micropuncture techniques to the study in young mammals of single nephron glomerular filtration rates and tubular function during early development have provided the first direct data on glomerulotubular balance during postnatal renal maturation. The technical limitations on such studies in the newborn kidney of mammals are considerable, but data of this type are essential to determine the type of glomerulotubular balance existing in superficial and deep nephrons during development and to define the factors regulating it.

Čapek, Dlouhá, and Kubát[81] described the results of micropuncture studies in 20- and 30-day-old rats in which they measured transit time (TT), resorption rate, intratubular pressures, GFR (total and individual), TF/p inulin, and length and inner diameter of proximal tubules. The intrinsic resorptive capacity increased with age (at 20 days $t_{1/2} = 13.6$ sec, at 30 days $t_{1/2} = 9.7$ sec) and TT decreased from 12 sec at 20 days to 9.2 sec at 30 days. In spite of the smaller proximal tubular volume, TT at 20 days was prolonged in comparison with adult rats and partly compensated for the lower intrinsic resorptive capacity. Consequently fractional resorption was not significantly different in the shorter and smaller young nephrons than in the adult nephrons. The authors did not give data on the absolute amount of sodium resorbed by the proximal tubules in the two groups.

Horster and Valtin,[25] employing micropuncture and clearance studies, have made a longitudinal study of postnatal development of renal function in the dog. They found that GFR of superficial nephrons increased from 3.2 nl/min at 21 days to 23.1 at 77 days. Despite this rise in filtered load, fractional resorption of sodium and water in superficial proximal tubules was constant and at the mature level from the onset of intratubular perfusion (see Fig. 3.2). Functional glomerulotubular balance was evident during the entire postnatal period, including the early period where there is disproportionate growth of tubular mass and volume with respect to glomerular volume.

Their data support the concept that renal maturation involves two growth phases: one representing cellular and anatomic maturation correcting nephron imbalance and heterogeneity reflecting differences in nephron age, the other involving proportionate increases in size and function during childhood growth. Functional glomerulotubular balance appears to be maintained in both phases, as judged by studies of single nephron function. Horster and Valtin postulated that changes in arterial plasma protein concentration, in filtration fraction, and in the hydrostatic pressure gradient between proximal tubule and peritubular capillary may interact to maintain glomerulotubular balance. The findings define for the first time some of the characteristics of the functional adaptations that maintain a glomerulotubular balance comparable to that of mature nephrons in the small-sized proximal tubules of the maturing nephrons.

The studies of Hayslett, Kashgarian, and Epstein[79] measuring the functional correlates of compensatory renal hypertrophy in mature rats revealed that following uninephrectomy tubular resorption of sodium was augmented as the filtration rate increased; this was associated with an increase of 17 percent in average diameter of proximal tubules. The fractional resorption of glomerular filtrate in the proximal and distal tubules of single nephrons remained the same, however, in the hypertrophied kidney with its fewer but larger nephrons as in the normal kidney.

Additional evidence that functional balance is maintained in the structurally enlarging nephron as it hypertrophies in response to contralateral nephrectomy is provided by Arrizurieta De Muchnik, Lipham, and Gottschalk.[82] In studies measuring changes in single nephron function and morphology utilizing techniques of micropuncture and microdissection in rats, these authors concluded that fractional resorption of sodium and water in normal and hypertrophied nephrons is similar and that the rates of resorption and delivery of fluid at any point along the hypertrophied nephron increase in proportion to the increase of filtration rate in its glomerulus. The mechanism whereby glomerulotubular balance is maintained in these situations of growth has yet to be defined.

In related studies Katz and Epstein[80] found that the increase in GFR outstripped the increase in size (weight) of the kidney during the period when the greatest increase in renal mass (and presumably growth activity) occurred—that is, 3 days to 2 to 3 weeks after nephrectomy. The progressive increase in GFR that occurs with compensatory hypertrophy may be analogous to the pattern of change in GFR relative to C_{PAH} and Tm_{PAH} in the neonatal period of infancy. Studies of the changes in GFR and RPF in rats and puppies in the neonatal period[24,25] showed that GFR increases more rapidly than RPF during the period of most vigorous postnatal growth.

The relevance of studies of changes in renal function during postnatal maturation of newborn and young animals to the situation in man is dependent on the degree to which the animal selected can be shown to warrant comparison with an equivalent stage in human development with respect to specific organ growth patterns.

Renal function in the neonatal rat and dog is not the most suitable model for comparison to the normal human newborn because formation of new nephrons continues postnatally in both. The 4- to 5-week-old animal would be more comparable to the human newborn because by then neogenesis has ceased. The use of young mammals thus requires careful selection of an appropriate model.

SUMMARY

Actual values for the major parameters of renal function change with growth as renal size increases with enlarging body mass. The rate of change is most rapid in the immediate postnatal period. By the fifth postnatal day GFR and RPF increase by 40 to 50 percent, reflecting a marked increase in renal blood flow as a result of changes in the distribution of cardiac output after removal of the placental circulation at birth. The rate of increase in actual values is most rapid in the first year of life, decreasing gradually thereafter in a pattern similar to that described for height and weight. Further increase stops concomitantly with the cessation of growth in lean body mass at the time of sexual maturation. Values for each discrete renal function when related to the surface area of the average normal adult (1.73 m² S.A.) are lowest at birth, values for GFR being 30 to 40 percent of those in adults and values for RPF and tubular secretory mass (Tm_{PAH} and $Tm_{GLUCOSE}$) being even lower (20 to 30 percent) when compared to adults.

The functional pattern of the newborn kidney is thus characterized by a relative preponderance of glomerular filtration per unit of renal blood flow and functioning tubular secretory mass. The morphologic findings are in agreement with the functional data. Both types of data suggest that this underdevelopment of tubular function relative to glomerular function is corrected by about the sixth month of postnatal life in man. Functional glomerulotubular balance comparable to that existing in mature kidneys apparently is achieved in the kidney early in the postnatal period.

The usual practice in reporting measurements of renal function in subjects of different ages and body size is to relate the actual value to 1.73 m² S.A. When viewed by S.A. standards, the values of GFR, RPF, and Tm_{PAH} and $Tm_{GLUCOSE}$ rise to levels comparable to those of adults by 2 to 3 years of age and remain within this range into adulthood. The range of normal values for specific renal functions in older children accordingly are similar to those for adults, though the data are somewhat limited in later childhood.

The physiologic significance of this observation is obscure. The stabilization of values at adult levels in early childhood when related to 1.73 m² S.A. may be associated with the relative constancy of the relation between the volume of extracellular fluid and lean body mass that exists after the first 6 months of life and persists until sexual maturation when sex-related differences are clearly apparent. The time at which values for renal function rise to adult levels (2 to 3 years) by surface area standards does not correlate with the time when cellular and functional evidences of immaturity disappear (6 months of age) and hence is not a true index to the time when this phase of renal maturation is completed. Values for discrete renal functions in subjects in the period before they have reached adult levels by surface area standards should be evaluated by comparison with the normal range for that age (from birth to 2 years of age), since they increase two to three times from the low levels at birth but do so at a changing rate.

The investigator who is interested in separating renal function changes resulting from cellular maturation from changes caused by adaptation and normal organ growth faces a complicated problem when dealing with the newly born subject. An obvious requirement is to define what we mean by renal functional maturation as distinct from changes caused by normal growth hypertrophy.

Renal maturation has been evaluated by at least two aspects measurable in early extrauterine life. These are cellular transport capacity (and the underlying enzyme activity) per unit of tubular tissue and anatomic maturity (dimensional heterogeneity). Both aspects are underdeveloped at birth by comparison with adult kidneys. Both appear to be corrected in the first few months of extrauterine life in man. Normal renal growth is presumably also responsible for the significant postnatal functional changes that occur as reflected in the rapid increase in values for GFR, RPF, and Tm_{PAH} and $Tm_{GLUCOSE}$ during this period. Both phenomena (cellular maturation and normal growth) contribute to the achievement of stable functional glomerulotubular balance that appears to be established in the first 6 months of postnatal life, along with the disappearance of anatomic immaturity and the evidences of reduced cellular transport capacity per unit of tubular mass.

These changes can be used to signal the end of true postnatal renal maturation. Considerable growth of nephrons has still to occur, however, before the final levels of renal function characteristic of the adult are achieved. The latter growth process should be looked upon as being analogous to "work hypertrophy" found in all forms of adaptive growth as defined by Goss[83] and exemplified most strikingly by the model of renal compensatory hypertrophy induced by uninephrectomy. Renal growth during infancy and childhood should be considered as another form of normal adaptive growth. This form occurs as a consequence of increasing functional demands imposed on the young subject's kidney in parallel with the increase in body size characterizing normal childhood growth. This type of adaptive renal growth would presumably be under the same controls regulating all normal childhood growth mechanisms and would be responsible for the increase in kidney size and in values for specific renal functions observed as the child matures to his adult size.

It would appear to be a developmental and physiologic misnomer to consider all of the functional changes that occur with growth up to the time when renal function per 1.73 m² S.A. stabilizes (2 to 3 years of age) at adult levels as the result of the process of renal maturation and to ascribe the remaining functional changes after this achievement to simple work hypertrophy physiologically comparable to that found in adults. The mechanisms responsible for maintenance of functional glomerulotubular balance during growth hypertrophy may differ in the child and the adult since the cellular mechanisms involved do differ quantitatively with age (see Chapter 5). If we consider the whole time period required for the development of adult values for renal function as a maturation process, it can be viewed as involving two integrated processes. True anatomic and cellular maturation would be limited to intrauterine life and the first few months of postnatal life. Renal growth hypertrophy would begin at birth and continue throughout childhood until final *functional* maturation takes place at puberty simultaneously with sexual maturation and the associated cessation in further lean body growth. This can be considered as the end point of maturation occurring by adaptive growth.

Chapter 4. Renal Function in the Postnatal Period

As we have seen, the kidney at term has already developed respectable functional capability. With the infant's assumption of extrauterine life, it must be ready to accept dependence on oral intake for fluids and nutrients as well as reliance on renal excretion for regulation of the proper volume and chemical composition of its body fluids. The efficiency with which its kidney carries out the numerous regulatory functions involved in achieving this autonomous stability has been extensively investigated. Several studies on aspects of discrete renal function will be examined in detail, including regulation of water and electrolyte balance. The functional competence of the newborn kidney is most clearly evident when the composition of the urine passed is examined with respect to constituents tested for by routine urinalysis.

COMPOSITION OF URINE DURING THE NEWBORN PERIOD

Urine passed in the first few days after birth is normally free of protein and sugar and shows a large range of values for pH (5.0 to 7.0) and specific gravity (60 to 600 mOsm/l). There has been some confusion in the older literature about the frequency of proteinuria in the newborn. Doxiadis, Goldfinch, and Cole[1] clarified part of this problem by calling attention to the fact that urates in urine of high concentration (a situation known to exist in the newborn in the first week of life) can give "false" positive tests for protein when chemical reagents consisting of strong acids are employed in testing for the presence of protein.

In a recent study using 20 percent sulfosalicylic acid to estimate urine protein quantitatively in prematures and newborns, Rhodes, Hammel, and Berman[2] reconfirmed the rarity of significant proteinuria (greater than 30 mg percent) even in the first few days of life. They found that 21 percent of a small group did show proteinuria ranging from a trace (10 mg percent) to 3+ (>100 mg percent) on the first day, but all specimens were negative by the fourth day of life. Proteinuria is thus not "physiologic" in the newborn any more than it is at any other age in childhood and the finding of protein in amounts above 30 mg percent should call for further study of the problem.

Randolph and Greenfield[3] have shown that transient proteinuria of 30 mg percent or more is sufficiently uncommon (6.3 percent) throughout childhood (3 weeks to 12 years) to make this finding an indication for further study. They found that the peak incidence of proteinuria, 14.8 percent, was reached during adolescence. Transitory glucosuria can also be found[2] in a small number of infants (24 percent) and the mechanism responsible is unknown. This disappears by the second postnatal week.

The urine passed by newborns is normally sterile and essentially free of leucocytes. Increased numbers of epithelial cells—both squamous and round—are found, however, in urines passed at birth.[2-6] These usually disappear during the first week. Female infants have greater numbers of squamous cells than males, which reflects vaginal sloughing of cells into the urine. Thus if total white cells in the urinary sediment are counted, the result will be meaningless in detecting true leucocyturia. Pryles[7] has recommended the use of suprapubic bladder aspiration to simplify detection of true urinary-tract infection and to avoid bacterial contamination and spurious leucocyturia in newborns.

Cruickshank and Edmond[6] have demonstrated, however, that sterile, normally voided "clean-catch" specimens can be obtained in male and female newborns by a careful clean-catch technique; the risk of the inherent dangers of bladder puncture[8] and catheterization can thus be minimized if the latter is used only in problem cases. These authors quantitated cellular elements as well and found that 96 percent of the specimens contained less than 3 leucocytes per cubic millimeter of urine. This agrees with the earlier, more extensive studies of Stansfeld and Webb[9] and Lincoln and Winberg,[4] who found that 98 percent of urine from newborn infants (both boys and girls) contained 10 or fewer leucocytes per cubic millimeter. A slightly larger number of leucocytes may be found in normally voided urines from girls, but these sex differences disappear if specimens are obtained after perineal cleansing or catheterization. The urine of newborns does not normally contain red blood cells or renal cellular casts. Quantitative standards for evaluation of urinary protein and cellular elements in infants and children can thus be equally well applied to the newborn.

RENAL REGULATION OF WATER METABOLISM IN INFANTS

Maintenance of the osmolar concentration of body fluids and volume of total body water within the narrow limits required for healthy normal growth is accomplished by the integration of complex renal and extra-renal factors. Of the nonrenal factors, the following are the most important: (1) volume and composition of daily intake; (2) integrity of hypothalamic-pituitary pathways for regulating thirst and secretion of antidiuretic hormone (ADH) as required by the infant's needs; and (3) the amount and type of daily extrarenal water and electrolyte expenditures (losses). No quantitative consideration of the effectiveness of renal regulation of water metabolism is possible without consideration of the requirements imposed on renal function by these extrarenal factors.

Urine volume in infants as in adults thus depends not only on the integrity of renal function but also on water intake, nonrenal water expenditures, and the renal solute load derived from dietary intake and catabolism. The minimal daily urine volume required to maintain water balance for any subject (that is, the obligatory urine volume) can be estimated if the daily renal solute load and renal solute concentrating capacity is known. The renal solute load is comprised of the excess electrolytes available (sodium, potassium, chloride, and phosphate) and the nonprotein nitrogen derived from protein catabolism, of which urea is the major end product. The level of daily intake of sodium, potassium, and chloride largely determines what the nonurea solute load will be, and the level of protein intake and state of nitrogen balance determines what the urea load presented to the kidneys will be.

The renal aspects of regulation of water balance in infants have been extensively studied. The physiologic mechanisms involved in this aspect of renal function have been greatly clarified by recent studies, and a brief summary taken from Pitts[10] seems appropriate here.

Mechanisms for Urine Concentration and Dilution

The proximal tubule resorbs the bulk (two-thirds) of the water and ions of glomerular filtrate isoosmotically. In contrast, the distal nephron (distal convoluted tubule and collecting duct) resorbs a small but variable fraction of filtrate (one-fifth to one-eighth) in a manner suited to the needs of the moment. The epithelium of the distal nephron can establish relatively high ion and osmolar concentration gradients between blood and urine, and its variable permeability to water is controlled by circulating antidiuretic hormone. In all portions of the nephron the resorption of water is passive and determined by osmotic forces created by the resorption of ions, among which the active resorption of sodium is the primary event. The ability to form concentrated urine is associated with the presence of loops of Henle interposed between proximal and distal segments of the renal tubule.

The site of final elaboration of urine (dilute or concentrated) is the distal nephron, where urine is concentrated by achieving osmotic equilibrium with the papillary interstitium. The active resorption of sodium (solute) without diffusion of water from the filtrate in the ascending limb of the loop of Henle creates osmolar hypertonicity in the medullary interstitium. As a result of the unique vertical hairpin structure of the loops of Henle (relative to the horizontal cortex) and vasa recta, a countercurrent mechanism is created that achieves increasing hypertonicity in the medullary interstitium starting from the corticomedullary junction and increasing progressively down to the tip of the papilla. The fluid entering the distal convoluted tubule is hypotonic to plasma. In water diuresis, it remains so as it flows along the distal tubule and collecting duct. In antidiuresis, it rapidly becomes isotonic as it flows through the distal tubule and hypertonic as it passes through the collecting ducts, which now serve as osmotic exchangers giving up water to the hypertonic medullary interstitium as they course from the cortex to the apex of the renal papillae. The maximal osmolar concentration attained in the final urine equals that existing in the medullary interstitium.

The major factors limiting the degree to which urine can be concentrated by countercurrent multiplication have been enumerated by Wirz, Hargitay, and Kuhn.[11] Hypertonicity of the medullary and papillary interstitium and urine is directly related to: (1) the total quantity of sodium pumped out of the ascending limbs of the loops of Henle per unit of time; (2) the magnitude of the gradient against which it is pumped; and (3) the length of the countercurrent multiplier loop. Hypertonicity of the interstitium and urine is inversely related (1) to the linear velocity of flow through the loops of Henle; and (2) to the cross-sectional area of the loops. Solute concentration is favored by the delivery of a relatively small volume of fluid from the proximal tubule into the loops of Henle, provided the volume is sufficient to deliver an adequate quantity of sodium to the "sodium pumps" of the cells lining the ascending loops. Reduction in GFR and slowing of the flow of fluid along the collecting ducts permits osmotic equilibration of urine and the hypertonic medullary and papillary interstitium even though the tubule is relatively impermeable to water. Under these conditions a hypertonic urine can be elaborated even in the absence of circulating ADH.[12]

The water which diffuses out of the descending limbs of Henle's loops and out of the collecting ducts, and the sodium pumped out of the ascending limbs of Henle's loops, are removed by blood perfusing the vasa recta of the medulla and papilla. The linear orientation of these vessels (parallel to the ascending and descending limbs of Henle's loops and the collecting ducts) allows them to serve as countercurrent exchangers, thereby reducing the loss of osmotically active solutes from the medulla and papilla while still providing an adequate blood supply.

In *osmotic diuresis,* in which the volume of fluid resorbed by the proximal tubules (fractional resorption) is reduced by the presence of a non-resorbable solute, the linear velocity of flow is reduced and the diameters of the loops of Henle are increased since resorption of fluid is decreased and intratubular pressure rises. Medullary and papillary hypertonicity is reduced. Two additional factors warrant mention here—medullary blood flow and ADH. An increase in medullary and papillary blood flow reduces the tissues' hypertonicity by washing out osmotically active solutes. Blood flow may well be increased in both water diuresis and osmotic diuresis; hence tissue hypertonicity is reduced. In antidiuresis ADH (1) reduces medullary blood flow via the vasa recta, and (2) increases the permeability of the collecting ducts to water and urea, permitting the attainment of more nearly perfect diffusion equilibrium.[10]

The mechanism of dilution has been less adequately described, but the essential facts are known. As mentioned earlier, during water diuresis the hypotonic fluid entering the distal convoluted tubules remains hypotonic during its passage along the distal tubule and collecting duct. Both segments are relatively impermeable to water in the absence of circulating ADH; hence osmotic equilibrium is not attained. The fact that the tubular fluid is hypotonic as it leaves the loops of Henle indicates that the pumps in the ascending limb continue to operate in water diuresis and maintain at least some degree of medullary and papillary hypertonicity. This concept has been verified directly by studies of renal tissue osmolality in water diuresis.[13]

Capacity of the Newborn to Concentrate Urine

The mean value for maximal urinary osmolar concentration achieved by newborn infants is about 600 to 700 mOsm/l, a value below that found under similar conditions of water deprivation in older infants and children ($+1,000$ mOsm/l) when they are ingesting normal protein intakes.[14–16] Infants can rapidly increase their renal concentrating capacity after birth, achieving or exceeding 1,000 mOsm/l by 1 to 2 months. The lower values for "total" urine osmolality at birth were originally attributed to immaturity of mechanisms for renal solute concentrations. The full significance of the finding of low values for urine solute concentration during postnatal growth has, however, only recently been appreciated.

The mechanisms involved in renal water conservation and excretion by the newborn infant's kidney are identical to those in the mature kidney. Certain special limitations are present, nevertheless, that are unique to the perinatal period and to the growing infant. These have now been clearly defined by numerous studies. A major factor is the relatively low GFR found in the newborn.[17,18] The rate of delivery of filtrate to the nephron is dependent on the glomerular filtration rate; consequently, GFR is a determinant of the maximal rate of excretion of electrolytes, solute, and water. A second factor is the striking anatomic and cellular underdevelopment of the tubular portions of the nephrons at birth. It can be assumed a priori that anatomic medullary immaturity accounts for some of the functional limitations. The osmolar gradient that could be achieved in the anatomically immature and relatively short medullary interstitium would not be comparable to that achieved in the large mature kidney with its fully developed nephrons and longer medulla.

Direct evidence in man to support this view is lacking, but it is available from animal studies where measurements of the magnitude of the osmolar gradient between cortex, medulla, and renal papilla have been made. The first investigations of this type were carried out in the author's laboratory on rabbits, newborn and during their first month of life.[19] As may be seen in Fig. 4.1A, the kidney of the newborn rabbit shows

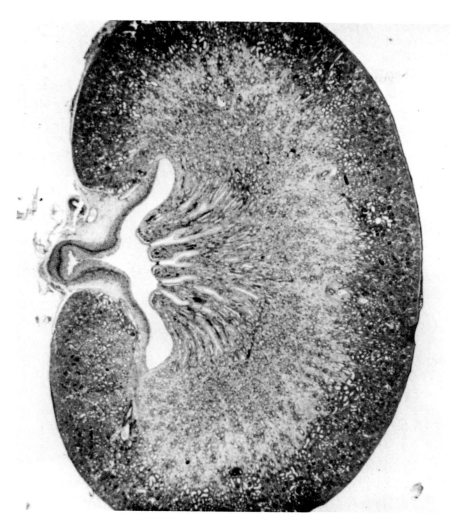

FIGURE 4.1A Kidney of the newborn rabbit in cross section, magnification x10. The renal papilla and medulla are very poorly developed.

a grossly evident lack of development of the inner medulla and the renal papilla. The whole medulla enlarges rapidly in the first week of life and the papilla becomes grossly prominent, increasing greatly in length when measured from the tip of the renal papilla to the corticomedullary junction (see Fig. 4.1B). The maximal urine solute concentration achieved

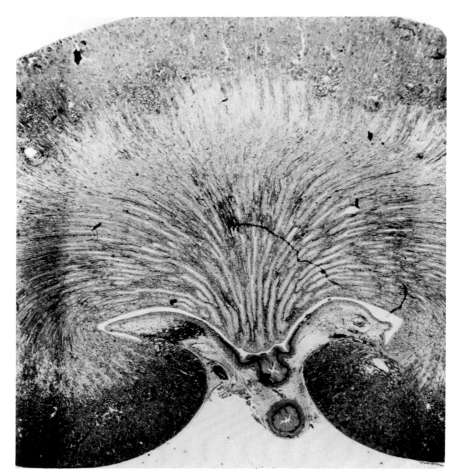

FIGURE 4.1B   Kidney of the week-old rabbit in cross section, magnification x10. The rapid growth of cortex and medulla is obvious when compared with the kidney of the newborn rabbit shown in Fig. 4.1A. The renal papilla and medulla have enlarged greatly and now resemble that seen in the adult kidney.

rises in the infant rabbit from low levels at birth (600 mOsm/l) to reach respectable (adult) levels by 3 weeks of age (2,000 mOsm/l).

The actual solute gradients found by direct measurement of cortex and medullary tissues in kidneys from infant rabbits deprived of food or fluid and given pitressin I-M eighteen hours before sacrifice followed a pattern of change that paralleled the anatomic and functional data, as shown in Fig. 4.2. The medullary-cortical sodium gradient rises postnatally to levels approaching values of mature rabbits by 6 weeks; urea, as would be expected, follows the same pattern (Table 4.1). These findings have been confirmed in rabbits[20] and in rats.[21] Anatomic examination revealed a considerable increase in the length and diameter of the loops of Henle and collecting ducts during this period. The medullary urea gradient was lower (as was the urinary urea concentration) in animals on low caloric diets that prevented normal growth. At 3 weeks of age the corticopapillary sodium gradient was, however, comparable to normals in spite of the runting (reduced rate of total body growth) that occurred. This would suggest that the rapid postnatal maturation

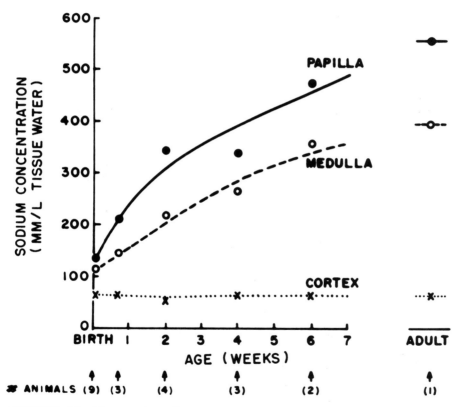

FIGURE 4.2 Changes in sodium concentration in the papilla, medulla, and cortex of the rabbit kidney during postnatal maturation. The gradient between papilla and cortex has increased from low levels at birth to that found in the adult kidney during hydropenia by 6 weeks after birth. Measurements were made on tissue fluid from pooled samples of serial sections of kidneys.

TABLE 4.1 Concentration of sodium and urea in kidney cortex and papilla of maturing rabbits

Age	No. of subjects	Sodium (mEq/l Tissue H_2O)			Urea (mm/l Tissue H_2O)		
		Cortex	Papilla	P/C[a]	Cortex	Papilla	P/C[a]
Newborn	9	61	137	2.2	24	115	4.8
5 days	3	63	211	3.3	45	319	7.1
13 days	4	57	345	6.1	25	345	13.8
28 days	3	64	340	5.3	22	367	16.7
42 days	2	68	477	7.0	23	488	26.6
Adult	1	64	560	8.7	14	512	36.6

[a] P/C = papilla/cortex ratio.

of the medulla is not solely dependent on the rate of general body growth in the postnatal period. Additional evidence that anatomic and functional maturation of the kidney can proceed independently of changes in dietary intake in weanling rats has been provided by Boss and his associates.[22]

A third factor involves postulated immaturity of the hypothalamic-posterior-pituitary pathways. Heller[23,24] has presented indirect evidence that the secretion of ADH is insufficient for the infant's needs and claims that the immature distal nephron has a low sensitivity to circulating ADH. The data presently available do not respond directly to the first proposition, since methods for measuring secretory rates of ADH are not presently available. There is some evidence to support the view that the newborn infant does not secrete sufficient ADH to meet the needs of hydropenia.[25,26] If the secretory capacity of the infant's posterior pituitary is limited at birth it would not be without parallel; the newborn parathyroid gland also appears to be relatively "quiescent" at birth, but it does show significant renal evidence of secretory activity by the third day of life.[27] If the secretory activity is limited at birth, this must be transitory; Calcagno, Rubin, and Weintraub[17] found no evidence of insufficient endogenous secretion of ADH in an 8-day-old premature infant who was exposed to osmotic loading during hydropenia.

There is indirect evidence that effective functional integrity of the hypothalamic-posterior-pituitary pathways exists in the newborn infant. Both full-term and premature newborn infants have the "ability" to elaborate a hypertonic urine (actually achieving an osmolar concentration twice that of plasma, 600 mOsm/l) since they do so within the first 24 hours after birth when no fluid intake is provided.[28] Smith and his colleagues[29] found evidence of a similar ability to concentrate urine in prematures fasted and thirsted for the first 2 to 3 days of life.

The pattern of change in urine osmolality observed in normal full-term newborns during the first week of life is shown in Fig. 4.3. The data on infants immediately after birth are from McCance and Widdowson[28] and the data from 1 to 6 days are from Heller.[23] Excretion of a dilute urine occurs after oral feedings begin, as can be seen by the fall in urine osmolality from the second day on. While this does not constitute direct evidence that ADH was responsible, it seems likely that the changes are mediated by alterations in endogenous secretion of ADH.

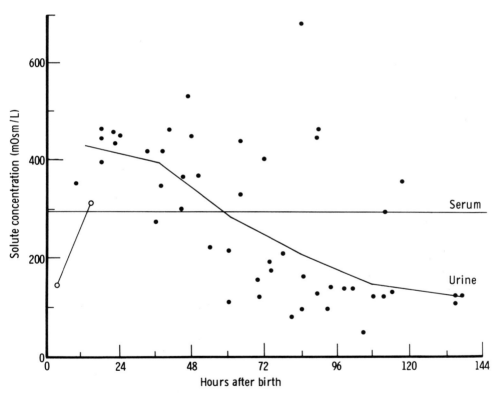

FIGURE 4.3   Average solute concentration in urines from normal newborns from birth to the sixth day of life. The data for the line describing changes in the first 24 hours (o——o) are taken from R. A. McCance and E. M. Widdowson.[28] (For details see Table 2.1.) The remaining data are reproduced from H. Heller[23] and represent urines from normal infants receiving normal fluid intakes.

The evidence of lack of responsiveness of the renal tubule of the infant to ADH is more difficult to assess. Ames[30] reported that infants of more than 3 days of age showed a definite antidiuretic response to exogenous pitressin given during substantial water diuresis, while infants of less than 3 days did not, although other physiologic evidences of pitressin effect were observed in these infants. Barnett and his co-workers[31] demonstrated conclusively that the 7-day-old infant's kidney responds promptly and appropriately with antidiuresis when given exogenous ADH during a water diuresis.

The maximal rate of tubular resorption of free water (Tm^cH_2O) measured during mannitol diuresis has been used as one means of estimating the magnitude of bulk flow of water across the distal nephrons and collecting ducts. It serves as one index of the permeability of the distal nephron and collecting duct to water. In normal adults Epstein and his colleagues[32] found the value for Tm^cH_2O varied from 5.3 to 7.2 ml/min. Measurements of Tm^cH_2O have been made in prematurely born infants 1 to 6 weeks of age by Calcagno, Rubin, and Weintraub[17] and lower values were found (3 to 5.2 ml/min) when corrected to 1.73 m^2 S.A. The values for GFR in these infants, however, were 30 to 50 percent of the value in adults; the lower values for Tm^cH_2O were largely attributable to this difference, since the range of values of the rate of Tm^cH_2O/C_{IN} was similar in infants and adults. The similarity of values for Tm^cH_2O in infants and adults when allowance is made for differences in GFR would suggest that comparable functional glomerulotubular balance exists in spite of the low GFR in the postnatal period, at least with respect to fractional water resorption.

The possibility that there is some decreased end-organ responsiveness to ADH in the newborn cannot be excluded. There is some support for this in the finding that urine osmotic U/P ratios were lower in the young infants during mannitol diuresis (about 2.5) than in adults (U/P ratio of about 4). Since exogenous ADH was given, the lower osmotic U/P ratios could not be attributed to insufficient circulating ADH. Calcagno's explanation for the decreased responsiveness is that it was related to decreased permeability (due to immaturity) of distal tubular epithelial cells to water. No directly relevant data are available, however, and other explanations are possible. Distal tubular resorption of sodium, which drives fluid movement, may be reduced and would favor the existence of a lower osmotic gradient in the renal medulla of the young infant. Another possibility is the consequences of anatomic underdevelopment of all of the medullary structures including the vasa recta and peritubular capillaries.

The studies reviewed have demonstrated that the concentrating mechanism matures rapidly (that is, achieves urine osmolality levels of 1,000 mOsm/l or higher) in the first months of postnatal life. While some limitation on renal osmolar concentrating ability in the newborn period is to be expected in the light of morphologic evidence of underdevelopment of the nephrons and medullary structures in the kidney, the maximal total osmolality in older infants differs from that in adults because of important nonrenal differences. These factors include the protein intake and the state of nitrogen balance and are often overlooked.

Extrarenal Factors Influencing Maximal Renal Concentrating Capacity

The ability of the kidney to concentrate urine has long been employed as a simple and informative test of renal function. In interpreting results of this test it is important to remember, however, that urea accounts for most of the urinary solute normally available for urine solute concentration in health. The evaluation of renal concentrating ability is valuable at any age only when the dietary protein intake and the state of nitrogen balance are known. Studies on normal infants[18] and adults[32] have shown that when protein intake is low or restricted the renal concentrating ability is reduced, whereas the ingestion of high-protein intakes or urea elevates the renal concentrating "ceiling."

Epstein and his co-workers[32] demonstrated that high intakes of protein or even urea alone increased the capacity of the adult's kidney for osmolal concentration and for maximal tubular resorption of free water during mannitol diuresis. Edelmann, Barnett, and Troupkou[18] demonstrated that the infant's concentrating capacity is similarly influenced by protein intake even in the first few weeks of life. They found that the mean maximal concentration in infants tested while on low-protein diets was 650 to 750 mOsm/l, while that achieved by the same infants on high-protein diets was 1,000 to 1,100 mOsm/l. The lower values of total osmolality were largely accounted for by the lower amounts of urea being excreted because of the low-protein intakes.[33] The concentration of nonurea solute was similar in infants on either diet. The higher values would thus be "normal" for infants on high-protein diets and the lower levels "normal" for the same infants if tested while on low-protein diets.

Similar differences would be expected between infants fed by the breast (1.7 percent protein) and with unmodified cow's milk (3.5 percent protein) because of the difference in protein intake. Such variations do not represent evidence of abnormal renal solute concentrating capacity since they result solely from the effects of alterations in rates of excretion of urea.

The higher rates of urea excretion in the infants on high-protein feedings did not increase renal water expenditures.[18] The mechanism of this "water sparing" effect of urea is of special interest to pediatricians. The increased urea production that occurs when high-protein diets are ingested does not increase obligatory urine volume or water needs, because the renal medulla "concentrates" urea to a greater degree when it is readily available. This has the effect of increasing the osmolar gradient in the medulla and thereby elevating the Tm^cH_2O and the ceiling for maximal achievable urine osmolality levels proportional to the increase in urea load. This holds true, however, only within fixed limits.[33] If the ingested urea load is excessive, urea will then act as an osmotic diuretic and lower urine solute concentration while augmenting urine volume.

Another unique aspect of the infant concerns the differences in nitrogen balance in the fasted infant as contrasted with the fasted adult. This is important because fluid restriction in infants also results in fasting. Measured nitrogen losses are lower in the fasting infant because urea production does not increase during starvation as it does in the adult.[34] The renal solute load thus may actually decrease during short periods of starvation in healthy infants because of their greater anabolic activity.

This has been strikingly demonstrated by Poláček and his associates,[16] who showed that infants 1 to 3 months old with water intakes reduced for twenty-four hours without a decrease in protein and solute intake (by feeding normal solids with half the usual water intake) were able to achieve total solute concentrations of 1,000 mOsm/l, comparable to results observed in older children and adults with twelve-hour fluid restriction (Fig. 4.4). Infants of the same age tested in the usual way, however (fasted and thirsted), all had lower "ceilings" (700 to 800 mOsm/l) which persisted throughout the first year of life.

Normal Values for Renal Concentrating Ability in Infants and Children

The normal mean value for maximal urinary solute concentration rises from a low value of 515 mOsm/l at 3 days of age to 663 mOsm/l at 6 days. It continues to rise in early infancy, reaching mean values of about 1,000 mOsm/l by 2 months if tested by the procedure of Poláček (Fig. 4.4). When all fluid intake is restricted and vasopressin adminis-

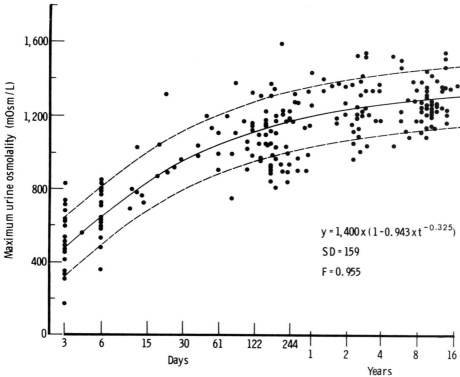

FIGURE 4.4   Relation of maximum urine osmolality to age in healthy infants and children. Maximum osmolality of urine samples in the course of 24-hour concentration test determined by means of double concentrated milk. Dotted lines indicate ±1 standard deviation. Logarithmic scale for age reproduced from E. Poláček et al.[16]

tered, the normal infant does not achieve a mean ceiling of 1,000 mOsm/l or higher until 2 years of age.[15,16] The mean values for the rest of childhood are only slightly above this level (mean value 1,075 mOsm/l, range 870 to 1,300 mOsm/l) if the test is performed under standardized conditions with overnight fluid restriction to subjects ingesting normal protein intakes.[35]

The equipment to measure solute concentration is not always available and specific gravity must then be employed. Edelmann and his colleagues[35] have compared the correlation between the two measurements in infants and children under standardized conditions and found that when the specific gravity was 1.027 or higher an osmolality of over 870 was assured. An osmolality of above 870 would be normal in all probability, since this represents the lower limit of the normal range. The elegantly simple test described by Poláček would appear to merit adoption as a routine procedure, whenever feasible, for formula-fed subjects. The results are more reproducible than those with fasting and thirsting alone or combined with parenteral administration of vasopressin as reported by Winberg.[15]

The feeding of concentrated formulas relatively high in protein could under certain conditions pose a threat to an infant's state of hydration. This danger would arise whenever the renal solute load requiring excretion during the test exceeded the supply of "free water" available for urine formation (that is, not required to meet nonrenal water expenditures) even in the presence of normal urinary solute concentration ability. In a classic study Darrow, Cooke, and Segar[36] demonstrated that when infants were in hot environments (ambient temperature above 70 to 75 F) a concentrated milk feeding as the sole source of fluid induced dehydration and azotemia in normal young infants. This risk would limit the use of Poláček's procedure in hot climates and in infants with renal disease associated with poor concentrating ability.

Capacity for Water Excretion

The newborn has a limited capacity for renal water excretion. The changes in renal response to water loads as the infant ages in the postnatal period have been studied by a number of workers.[17,24,26,30,31] The rapidity with which limitations present at birth are corrected in the first two weeks of life was elegantly demonstrated by the studies of Ames,[30] who measured the time of appearance and rate of increase in urine volume and fall in urinary specific gravity observed in the two-hour period after administration of a water load.

She demonstrated that the newborn had a very limited water diuresis (15 percent of load excreted by two hours) in response to orally and intravenously administered water loads (Fig. 4.5). There was a progressive increase in the rapidity with which urine volume rose in infants tested during the first two weeks after birth such that infants older than 2 weeks of age responded in a manner similar to that found in adults (that is, 100 percent of load excreted by two hours). There was a slight delay (about 20 minutes) in the onset of diuresis when water was ingested orally rather than intravenously, but the differences in rate of increase in urine flow between infants less than 3 days old and those

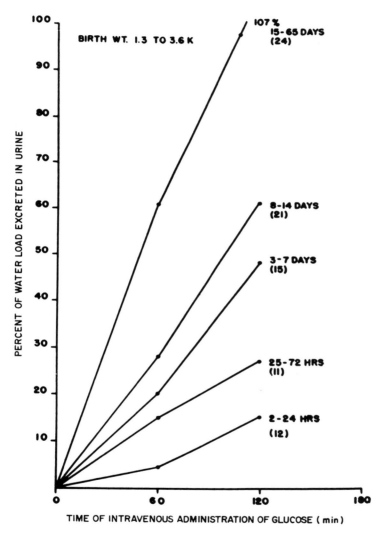

FIGURE 4.5 Comparison of water excreted by various age groups following intravenous administration of 2.5 percent glucose as 30 cc/kg body weight given at approximately —10 to 0 min. Figures in parentheses indicate number of patients in each group. (From R. G. Ames.[30])

older did not disappear when water was administered intravenously to both groups of subjects. The importance of the effect of the route of fluid administration on diuretic response has been documented by Hoy,[37] who changed the slow and moderate renal response observed when newborn rats were given oral water and salt loads to a prompt and significant diuresis when the intravenous route was used.

Ames's interesting and important observations as depicted in Fig. 4.5 show how rapidly increased renal functional capacity (for water diuresis) can develop in the postnatal period. Calculation of the proportion of filtered water excreted when the infants 1 to 14 days old achieved maximal urine volumes in her studies[30] and those of Barnett and his associates[31] reveals that urine volumes represented 20 to 30 percent of their GFR; even the 1-day-old infants studied by Ames excreted urine volumes representing 20 to 25 percent of their GFR. This value indicates that the overall capacity of the immature nephrons for fractional excretion of filtered water is similar to, if not greater than, that found in older subjects and adults.

Since the ability of the youngest infants to dilute urine is not impaired,[17,31] the major limiting factor affecting the newborn infant's rate of water diuresis is again found to be the lower rate of GFR. It is of interest that Ames found no apparent differences in diuretic response or rate of increase in urine volume between prematures and full-term infants of comparable postnatal age. The differences between newborn and older infants appear to be largely dependent on the low GFR that exists at birth, and the increased capacity observed with aging correlates well with the postnatal increase in GFR.

RENAL SODIUM EXCRETION

The tendency of infants temporarily to retain sodium ingested in excess of growth requirements is well recognized, especially in the neonatal period. In young infants sudden increases in intakes of salt, as a result of formula changes or parenteral administration beyond the amounts required to replace normal expenditures and supply needs for growth, will be temporarily retained. This excess can lead to acute expansion of the extracellular fluid volume with transitory weight gain and at times edema[38]—even, if water intake is inadequate, to hypernatremia.[39] The retention of sodium under these conditions has been ascribed to renal immaturity.

Dean and McCance[40] were the first to study renal sodium excretion in young subjects. They found that infants had a reduced ability to excrete sodium loads (hypertonic saline intravenously) when compared with adults who were given equivalent sodium loads calculated on the basis of surface area. While this observation was initially of great interest, it is now less surprising in the light of the other well-recognized differences in surface area per unit of body mass, volume of extracellular fluid, total body water, and GFR in infancy and adulthood (see Chapter 3). It no longer seems appropriate to employ such comparative "equal load studies" in young and old subjects measuring rates of renal sodium excretion if we wish to define the specific physiologic extra- and intrarenal mechanisms controlling sodium excretion in the infant from the developmental standpoint.

Functional Organization of Proximal and Distal Tubular Electrolyte Transport

Giebisch[41] has summarized the recent morphologic and electrophysiologic evidence that suggests there are differences in the functional organization of proximal and distal tubular electrolyte transport. The proximal tubular cell model he proposes (Fig. 4.6) consists of two parallel compart-

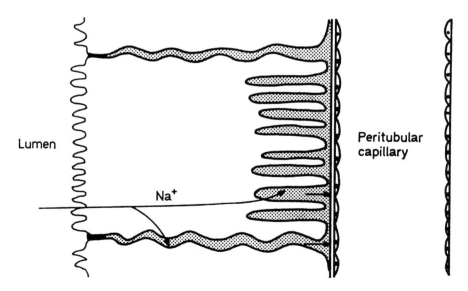

FIGURE 4.6 Schematic presentation of some properties of single proximal tubule cells. (From G. Giebisch.[41])

ments that comprise the intraepithelial fluid pathway. In addition to the classic transcellular route of ion movement from lumen to peritubular capillary in the basal cell membrane, there are functionally important low-resistance extracellular shunt pathways between cells connecting the tubular lumen with the peritubular fluid. As shown in Fig. 4.6, the tubular cell has a luminal and peritubular cell membrane. Adjacent cells are connected apically by tight junctions. These are particularly short in the proximal tubule epithelium and considerably more prominent in the distal tubule.

The intracellular space may be much more complex than the single compartment shown here. The tight junction and the intercellular space are thought to be the extracellular shunt pathways. As indicated by the black arrow, sodium is thought to be transported from the cell interior into the interspaces with water following passively across the cell membrane. It is well established that a very large fraction of the glomerular filtrate is resorbed along the proximal tubule, and the main primary transport process in this operation is the active transfer of sodium out of the tubular lumen into the peritubular fluid. It has been shown in microperfusion studies that back flux of sodium from the peritubular compartment to the lumen is extensive.

A number of authors[42-44] have shown that factors affecting peritubular capillary fluid resorption can modify proximal net fluid and sodium transport. These include the hydrostatic pressure and colloid osmotic pressure of the fluid perfusing the proximal tubule. While the precise underlying mechanisms are not yet clear, the demonstration that changes in peritubular filtration pressure, in peritubular blood flow, and in peritubular oncotic pressure affect resorptive proximal net sodium transport is of great importance. The role of intraepithelial transport pathways in these functional changes will require further study. The proposed cell model has many functional consequences that will necessitate a reevaluation of our notions of some active transport patterns, and the interested reader should consult the stimulating report by Giebisch.[41]

The transport properties of the distal tubule and collecting ducts reveal certain differences from those of the proximal tubule, especially in the transport of potassium. The sodium concentration normally declines along the distal tubule while that of potassium increases, whereas potassium concentration decreases along the proximal tubule. The mechanism responsible for the apparent secretion of potassium by the distal tubule and collecting duct is still a matter of controversy, and the "classical" distal sodium-potassium-hydrogen exchange model is undergoing reevaluation. Giebisch has proposed a cell model that does not include a tightly coupled sodium-potassium exchange mechanism. He also omits a direct pump-related competition between potassium and hydrogen secretion. It should be abundantly clear that there are still gaps concerning numerous aspects of the functional organization of proximal and distal tubular cells. The study of single-nephron function in the developing nephron may provide useful data to fill the gaps in our knowledge and to complement that obtained by more traditional experiments using "mature nephrons."

Factors Regulating Renal Sodium Excretion

A higher rate of sodium excretion can be attained by increasing filtered load (by raising GFR and/or plasma sodium level) without increasing net tubular resorption thus lowering fractional sodium resorption, or directly by decreasing rate of tubular resorption without a change in filtered load to lower fractional sodium resorption. It would appear that the level of GFR may play an important role in determining the rate of sodium excretion in infants. Because of the large volume of glomerular filtrate formed daily (180 liters) in the adult, large amounts of sodium can be removed by small changes (1 to 2 percent) in fractional resorption. A decrease of 1 percent in fractional resorption of sodium with GFR and plasma level of sodium remaining constant would result in the excretion over a 24-hour period of 252 mEq of sodium (1 percent of Na in 180 liters of filtrate). This is equivalent to 15 grams of salt, a large intake even for an adult.

In the newborn infant with a GFR 30 to 50 percent that of the adult per 1.73 m² S.A., this same mechanism operating similarly would be less effective. The lower GFR relative to his larger extracellular fluid volume could thus appear to predispose the infant to sodium retention; this could be interpreted teleologically as having survival value for the newly born infant. It seems probable that there is larger filtration volume per nephron in the infant kidney than in the mature kidney. If this is demonstrated to exist, any further increase in filtration load of sodium (by either increase in GFR or elevation of serum sodium level) would exaggerate this relative glomerular preponderance and might facilitate sodium excretion by decreased fractional resorption of filtered sodium. There may, however, be no limitation on the infant's capacity for maintaining glomerulotubular balance while preserving its capacity to increase renal sodium excretion under stress, even with the differences in GFR when compared with the adult.

Edelmann[45] has measured the renal naturetic response of the newborn piglet to intravenous isotonic saline and observed that there is a significant and prompt increase in the rate of sodium excretion associated with a decrease in fractional resorption of filtered sodium from values of 98 to 99 percent in the control period to values as low as 85 percent of the filtered load under maximal naturesis. The response in terms of fractional rate of sodium excretion was qualitatively similar to that seen in mature animals after expansion of vascular volume. The study was not designed to provide information about the intrarenal changes responsible for the calculated decrease in fractional sodium resorption observed.

Expansion of vascular or extracellular fluid volume in dogs[46] and rats[47] is associated with a decrease in fractional resorption of filtered sodium. The mechanism responsible remains under study. Knowledge of how these intrarenal factors controlling sodium excretion operate in the immature kidney is, however, almost nonexistent.

As pointed out above, one pathway for transtubular movement of sodium occurs via extracellular routes[13] involving spaces between the renal tubular cells distal to the junctional complexes which connect neighboring cells at their luminal surface junctions, and these may not act as a perfect seal. The possibility exists that in the immature nephron there is a less effective "seal" and in consequence the transepithelial sodium pump operates less effectively to move sodium to the peritubular space because of greater retrograde flux back into the tubular lumen. There may be less effective removal of sodium extruded into the peritubular space. The contribution of the various factors influencing net tubular transport of sodium from the tubular lumen into the peritubular compartment have yet to be defined in the immature kidney.

Renal sodium excretion is also under the hormonal control of aldosterone. There is no evidence to suggest that the nephron in the normal newborn is not responsive to aldosterone. In my own group[48] we have shown that the kidney in the 6-day-old infant responds to exogenous aldosterone in a normal manner. The rate of sodium excretion decreases without a change in filtered load, indicating that there is increased fractional resorption of filtered sodium in response to aldosterone administration.

In summary, present evidence (clinical and physiologic) would indicate that except for the recognized limitations imposed by a relatively low GFR the renal mechanisms for sodium excretion appear to be operating quite effectively in the newborn. More data are needed before we can define any differences in intrarenal mechanisms regulating renal handling of sodium that can be truly ascribed to immaturity.

RENAL ACID-BASE REGULATION

The newborn infant has been shown to have a limited capacity for renal elimination of hydrogen ions when compared with the adult. While this limitation reflects the functional and anatomic immaturity already discussed, nonrenal factors also are important. The adjustment from intrauterine life to extrauterine existence imposes new functional demands upon the kidney, which now must assume responsibility for regulation of the infant's acid-base balance. In order to respond fully to the demands imposed by the new circumstances of extrauterine life with oral milk feedings, time will be required to allow growth of glomeruli and nephrons and cellular adaptations to correct existing limitations. It is well known that adults given acute loads of "fixed acid" (that is, NH_4Cl loads) require three to five days to achieve maximal rates of excretion of titratable acid and ammonia and thus maximal conservation of "fixed base" to preserve body buffer stores.

Resorption of Bicarbonate

A brief review taken from Pitts[49] of the normal mechanisms responsible for renal bicarbonate resorption and hydrogen ion excretion is useful before considering the developmental aspects. A proximal tubular mechanism is specialized to resorb the bulk of the filtered bicarbonate from tubular urine against a relatively low gradient. Sodium and bicarbonate ions enter the proximal tubular lumen in the glomerular filtrate. Sodium ions passively diffuse into the tubular cells down a concentration and electrical gradient and are actively extruded into the peritubular fluid by a secretory pump which maintains intracellular sodium concentration at a low value. The tubular secretion of hydrogen ions in the reverse direction to the movement of sodium ions is active, requiring a secretory pump, and is the key mechanism underlying the resorption of bicarbonate.

Hydrogen ions move from the interior of the cell to the tubular lumen against an electrical gradient in exchange for sodium ions. They then associate with bicarbonate ions to form carbonic acid, which decomposes into carbon dioxide and water. The carbon dioxide diffuses into the cell, where it undergoes hydration to form carbonic acid—a reaction which is catalyzed by carbonic anhydrase. Subsequent dissociation provides hydrogen ions which are available for exchange for sodium ions moving across the luminal membrane and bicarbonate ions which diffuse down a potential gradient into the peritubular fluid and into the peritubular capillaries.

Two independent mechanisms involved in bicarbonate resorption have been identified: (1) a carbonic-anhydrase-dependent mechanism, the enzyme having a cellular and luminal action;[50,51] and (2) a pCO_2-dependent mechanism which does not require cellular activity of carbonic anhydrase and is mediated by uncatalyzed hydration of CO_2.[52] The major difference between the proximal and distal tubular mechanisms is that the dehydration of the carbonic acid is catalyzed in the proximal tubule and uncatalyzed in the distal tubule.

The presence of carbonic anhydrase on the brush border of proximal tubules no doubt facilitates the bulk resorption of bicarbonate because it reduces by a factor of ten the gradient against which hydrogen ions must be secreted and correspondingly reduces the energy cost of bicarbonate conservation. The mechanisms for the resorption of bicarbonate in distal tubules and collecting ducts are qualitatively the same as in proximal tubules, but the former differ quantitatively in two respects. First, together they account for only 10 percent of the total bicarbonate resorption. Second, they are capable of salvaging essentially all of the bicarbonate remaining in the tubular fluid when the plasma concentration is normal or low.

To accomplish this latter end, the collecting ducts, specifically, must be able to secrete hydrogen ions against much steeper gradients than either proximal or distal tubules. Also, sodium ions may have to be pumped from lumen into cells to accomplish their nearly complete removal in states of sodium depletion. Accordingly, a more tightly coupled hydrogen-sodium exchange pump may be present in the collecting ducts. The limiting gradient against which hydrogen ions can be pumped in forming urine of maximum acidity is about 1,000:1, a value which relates blood pH of 7.4 to urine pH of 4.4. Since final acidification of the urine is accomplished in the collecting ducts, maximal gradients are developed in this portion of the nephron. The low rate of bicarbonate transport and the capacity to develop a steep hydrogen ion gradient makes luminal carbonic anhydrase unnecessary in the distal tubule and collecting ducts.[49]

The gross characteristics of the processes of renal resorption and excretion of bicarbonate in man resemble those of a T_m-limited process. All of the bicarbonate filtered is resorbed in the normal human subject until the plasma level attains a value of 26 to 28 mm/l—the so-called renal bicarbonate threshold. If the plasma level is elevated beyond this by bicarbonate infusion, a limited amount of bicarbonate equal to 2.8 mm/100 ml or 28 mm/1 of glomerular filtrate is resorbed. All bicarbonate filtered in excess of this quantity is excreted in the urine.

The renal bicarbonate threshold in the dog and man is by no means an unvarying constant. At least four factors influence it: (1) changes in the CO_2 tension of arterial blood; (2) variations in the body store of potassium; (3) variations in the plasma level of chloride; and (4) variations in the secretion of adrenal cortical hormones. A recent report by Purkerson and his associates[53] has shown that the bicarbonate T_m varies also with the GFR and with changes in extracellular fluid volume. Thus bicarbonate resorption, in common with sodium resorption, is characterized by glomerulotubular balance. These two spatially separated structures, the proximal tubules and distal nephrons and collecting ducts, may be involved separately or together in situations characterized by renal bicarbonate wasting (or renal tubular acidosis).

In view of the quantitative differences in bicarbonate resorption in proximal and distal tubules, some investigators[54,55] have proposed that two clinical forms of renal tubular acidosis (Types I and II) be distinguished as separate entities depending on whether they represent (1) disturbances of mechanisms controlling the threshold or rate of tubular resorption of bicarbonate representing Type I and designated as proximal[54] or rate defects[55] causing renal tubular acidosis (RTA), or (2) inability to establish or maintain normal pH gradients between blood and distal tubular fluid representing classical or Type II RTA and designated as distal[54] or gradient[55] defects causing RTA. The physiologic basis for the separation seems evident and both distinctions possess some clinical value.

Bicarbonate Resorption in Infants

Tudvad, McNamara, and Barnett[56] examined the renal bicarbonate excretion in premature infants 8 to 37 days of age and found the mean value of the renal bicarbonate threshold (level of serum bicarbonate at which bicarbonate excretion appears in urine) to be 22 to 24 mMoles/l. This is slightly lower than the threshold of 24 to 26 mMoles/l in normal adults found by Pitts, Ayer, and Schiess.[50] However, the maximal rate of bicarbonate resorption (Tm_{HCO_3}), 2.5 to 2.6 mMoles/l/min, was quite close to the range found in adults, 2.6 to 2.9 mMoles/l/min. Edelmann and his co-workers[57] measured renal bicarbonate resorption in full-term infants from 1 to 16 months of age and found a value for the renal threshold (21.5 to 22.5 mMoles/l) similar to that found in premature infants by Tudvad, while the value for Tm_{HCO_3} (2.6 to 2.9 mMoles/l) was now similar to that of adults.

If the results of Tudvad and his group are representative of the neonatal full-term infant, Edelmann's data indicate that the renal tubular capacity for bicarbonate resorption in infants is functionally comparable to that of adults by 1 to 2 months of age. A slightly lower renal threshold for bicarbonate persists, however, throughout the first year of life. This lower threshold cannot be accounted for by limitation in overall renal capacity for bicarbonate resorption, since the value for bicarbonate Tm in infants is as high as that in adults. Edelmann suggested that it could be caused by persistent functional heterogeneity of nephrons.

The physiologic significance of the infant's lower renal threshold in the first year of life is somewhat obscure. It could be a factor contributing to the low CO_2 content of arterialized capillary blood found[58] in infants between 3 months and 2 years (21.1 ± 1.9 mMoles/l), since the bicarbonate level in plasma is determined by the renal "threshold." It could also be a consequence of a general systemic process rather than the cause of the lower blood bicarbonate concentration. Since the Tm_{HCO_3} in infants over 1 month of age is similar to that of older children, there is no evidence to indicate that there is a limitation in rate of overall renal capacity for bicarbonate resorption.

Excretion of Hydrogen Ions in Infants

Renal excretion of hydrogen ions is responsible normally for restoration of normal concentrations of buffer base (bicarbonate) from body stores utilized to neutralize strong acids, such as sulfuric and phosphoric, arising from the metabolism of proteins and phospholipids. They are transported by the kidney as neutral salts. There are two renal mechanisms involved in hydrogen ion excretion by the kidney: (1) urinary acidification, which results in the removal of nonvolatile acids as free acid or acid salts (measured as titratable acidity and organic acids); and (2) ammonium excretion by the removal of H+ ions via combination with ammonia secreted by the tubules to form neutral ammonium salts in the tubular lumen. These two renal mechanisms are both operating effectively even in newborn infants.

The initial rate of excretion is somewhat limited, but the rapidity with which postnatal adaptation occurs in the infant's renal mechanisms of acidification to meet the requirements of extrauterine life has been documented by Edelmann.[45] The daily urine pH in the first two weeks of life in premature infants receiving normal diets was measured; all infants achieved urine pH values below 5.4 by the eighth day of life, and some values below pH 5.0 were observed in the second week.

The quantitative aspects of renal acid excretion during growth have been well documented by Peonides, Levin, and Young[59] and more recently by Edelmann and his associates,[57,60] by observing the renal response of subjects at different ages to ammonium chloride loads. The former group evaluated the response of infants 2 to 12 months of age and older subjects (1 to 16 years) after three days of orally administered NH_4Cl (72 to 96 mEq/day/m² S.A.). They found the mean and range of values for total hydrogen ion excretion and for titratable acid (TA) and ammonium excretion to be similar in both age groups (see Table 4.2) and comparable to levels achieved by adults.

The Edelmann group studied the response of milk formula-fed infants 1 to 16 months of age to a single dose of NH_4Cl (75 mEq/m² S.A.) and found no evidence of a limitation in capacity for renal acidification between infants 1 to 3 months of age and those 3 to 16 months of age when differences resulting from GFR were accounted for. The ability of both groups of infants to acidify urine was similar (mean urine pH 4.9) and also comparable to that of subjects 7 to 12 years of age (mean urine pH also 4.9).

The normal values and ranges for the rate of total H+ excretion (sum of $TA + NH_4$/uEq/min/1.73 m² S.A.) in infants and children under the test conditions described are shown in Table 4.2. Infants had higher rates of excretion of TA and lower rates of NH_4 excretion than children, but this could be accounted for by the higher rates of excretion of phosphate arising from the infants' higher dietary intakes of phosphate.[61] There were no significant age-related differences in rates for renal ammonia excretion, if variations in GFR were accounted for. These studies have clearly shown that after the first few weeks of life the renal capacity

TABLE 4.2 Renal acid excretion of normal infants and children after NH_4Cl ingestion

	No. of subjects	Age	pH	Urine H$^+$	TA	NH$_4$	Serum (CO$_2$ mMol/l)
				(uEq/min/1.73 m^2 S.A.)			
Mean	12[a]	2–12 months		97.0	42.5	54.4	16.6
Range			4.8–5.8	67–172	21–72	26–100	11–20
Mean	14[a]	1–16 years		95.1	30.2	64.5	18.2
Range			4.7–5.6	62–165	14–54	46–111	14.0–21.4
Mean	11[b]	1–16 months	4.9	119	62	57	17.1
S.E.			±0.03	±9.2	±4.9	±4.3	±0.43
Mean	10[c]	7–12 years	4.9	130	50	80	18.5
S.E.			±0.06	±4.5	±3.1	±3.7	±0.66

[a] After three days' ingestion of 72 to 96 mEq NH_4Cl/m^2 surface area. (From A. Peonides, B. Levin, and W. F. Young.[59])

[b] Five to six hours after ingestion of 75 mEq NH_4Cl/m^2 surface area. (From C. M. Edelmann, Jr. et al.[57])

[c] Five to six hours after ingestion of 150 mEq NH_4Cl/m^2 surface area. (From C. M. Edelmann, Jr. et al.[57])

of infants to excrete hydrogen ion compares quite favorably with that of children and adults if allowances are made for differences in GFR.

Relation between Dietary Acid Load and Renal Acid Excretion

The rate of renal hydrogen ion excretion in infants varies depending on the diet they are ingesting, as it does at all ages.[62] The rate is higher and the urinary pH is lower in cow's-milk-fed infants than in breast-fed infants.[63] The rate of phosphate excretion is lower in breast-fed infants because the dietary intake is low and retention high. The low rate of renal PO_4 excretion limits the amount of urinary buffer (primarily PO_4) available for excretion as titratable acid and it limits the infant's capacity to excrete urines of low pH with a high titratable acidity, especially when tested by an acute NH_4Cl load. Ammonia secretion accounts for the major proportion of hydrogen ion excreted by breast-fed infants.[63] It is thus important to consider diet as well as age when evaluating the infant's capacity for urinary acidification.

The studies of Hatemi and McCance[64] have called attention to the physiologic normality of the observation that the breast-fed infant does not achieve as low a urinary pH under stress of an acid load as does the infant fed on cow's milk. They also demonstrated that orally administered loads of neutral phosphate (7 gm/kg/day) given to normal 7-day-old breast-fed infants raised their rate of titratable acid excretion and lowered the mean values for urine pH achieved after NH_4Cl loads. Calculations of their data reveal, however, that the actual rate of total hydrogen ion excretion per day in these phosphate-loaded infants and their net endogenous acid-base balance were not altered. This would be the expected normal renal response, since the administration of neutral inorganic phosphate would not change the infant's net load of hydrogen ion generated from endogenous and exogenous sources. The administration of more urinary buffer as neutral phosphate did, however, result in lower urine pH and increased titratable acidity in urine. It does not seem fitting to attribute to renal immaturity differences in renal hydrogen ion excretion that can be related to dietary intake.

More impressive from the developmental standpoint is the fact that infants on cow's-milk feedings excrete more renal acid than breast-fed infants of equal age. This provides evidence that the infant's kidney has the capacity to show adaptation to its renal "work loads" in a manner qualitatively similar to the mature kidney.

RENAL EXCRETION OF PHOSPHATE

Phosphate is involved in diverse essential metabolic processes in the body. Calcium phosphate is a major constituent of bone, and uptake and release of both elements occur simultaneously and continuously in skeletal tissues. Organic phosphate complexes play a key role in many vital energy transformations in cell metabolism. Inorganic phosphate provides the major readily available buffer component in urine and thus contributes importantly to the maintenance of normal acid-base balance in the body.

Plasma concentration is regulated by the kidney and it is influenced by hormonal factors that vary depending on the requirements for bone and organ cellular repair and growth.[65] The level is higher in utero and in early infancy than it is in children and adults. The adult in balance retains little phosphate and excretes, largely in urine, the same amount of phosphate that is ingested daily. After birth the infant kidney must rapidly develop the renal capacity to handle exogenous PO_4 requiring excretion each day at rates that prevent abnormal elevation of the plasma PO_4 levels. The adaptation from the controlled steady state of transplacental phosphate intake in intrauterine life to the repetitive and transitory elevations in serum PO_4 concentration that occur when the phosphate intake is provided by milk feedings requires (1) maturation of renal mechanisms for excretion, and (2) increased secretory activity of the parathyroid glands.

The serum phosphate level in newborns rises within the first 24 hours after birth and continues to rise, especially in infants receiving cow's-milk formulas, reaching a plateau level between the first and second weeks of the postnatal period.[27] The hyperphosphatemia then gradually subsides toward levels characteristic of infancy. The serum calcium level tends to change in a manner reciprocal to that of phosphate. When hyperphosphatemia persists, the disturbance in calcium and phosphate balance is severe enough to cause transitory hypocalcemia and convulsions (neonatal tetany) that respond promptly to measures that elevate serum calcium levels and depress serum phosphate levels.[66]

The hyperphosphatemia has been implicated as a factor of importance in the development of hypocalcemic tetany of the newborn.[67] Transient hyperphosphatemia has been attributed to the relatively high phosphate intake of cow's-milk-fed neonates[66] and to renal immaturity involving low GFR[68] and functional underdevelopment of renal tubular epithelium.[69] Limited secretory capacity of the neonate's parathyroid gland has also been proposed.[67] A brief review of the renal mechanisms regulating normal phosphate excretion may be useful before the role of renal immaturity is reviewed.

Mechanisms of Phosphate Excretion

The tubular mechanism of phosphate resorption[70] has the characteristics of a Tm-limited mechanism and is similar in many respects to that which reabsorbs glucose, with at least two important differences.

(1) The Tm for glucose is set so high that it is never exceeded under normal conditions, and consequently renal excretion of glucose plays no role in regulating the normal plasma glucose concentration. The Tm for phosphate, in contrast, is maintained at a level such that a slight increase or decrease in plasma concentration changes the rate of excretion and accordingly the kidney does participate actively in regulation of the plasma concentration.

(2) The Tm for phosphate is not "remarkably stable" from day to day, as is the case for glucose, but varies—at times significantly—depending on body stores of phosphate and circulating levels of certain hor-

mones especially that of the parathyroid gland. The rate of phosphate excretion (phosphate clearance, C_{PO_4}) is dependent on the filtered load of phosphate (GFR $\times$ plasma PO_4) and the Tm_{PO_4}. A change in the value of C_{PO_4} can result from a change in GFR or plasma level of phosphate. Factors decreasing Tm_{PO_4} include parathyroid hormone, vitamin D and cortisone, saturation of glucose resorption, and infusion of calcium. Parathyroid hormone can also increase PO_4 excretion by increasing plasma PO_4 concentration. Metabolic acidosis does not alter Tm_{PO_4}, but increases PO_4 excretion indirectly by elevation of the serum PO_4 level because of mobilization of bone and tissue stores of phosphate.

Mechanisms Regulating Renal Phosphate Excretion in the Newborn

My own group's examination of the renal mechanisms involved in PO_4 excretion in infants in the newborn period[68] demonstrated that all of the normal renal mechanisms were operative in newborn infants, but the low GFR was again found to be a major factor limiting their effectiveness. As shown in Table 4.3, we demonstrated that newborn infants receiving cow's-milk formulas were excreting phosphate at rates comparable to adults, but required higher plasma levels of PO_4 to do so. Studying the renal response of newborn infants to acute phosphate loads demonstrated that a maximal rate of phosphate excretion (Tm_{PO_4}) was evident. Changes in Tm_{PO_4} were evoked in response to alterations in phosphate absorption in the gut. Reduction in dietary phosphate resulted in decreased phosphate excretion associated with elevation in Tm_{PO_4} while GFR and serum phosphate concentration were unchanged. It was also shown that the fractional excretion of filtered phosphate (C_{PO_4}/C_{IN}) in the infants ingesting cow's milk (high-phosphate intake) was comparable to that found in normal children and adults. These changes in phosphate excretion could have been partly mediated by altered endogenous parathyroid secretory activity, since it was also demonstrated that 5- to 14-day-old infants exhibited a significant phosphaturic effect when given exogenous parathyroid intravenously.

Connelly, Crawford, and Watson[27] subsequently showed that 1- and 3-day-old newborn infants also exhibit a renal phosphaturic effect when given exogenous parathyroid hormone, although the response in the 1-day-old infant was much reduced in comparison to that observed in the 3-day-old infant. They interpreted their data as suggesting that the kidney of the 1-day-old newborn is less sensitive to the renal effects of parathyroid hormone. An alternative explanation could be that the low

TABLE 4.3 Comparison of renal excretion of phosphate at endogenous serum phosphate concentrations in infants, children, and adults (from W. W. McCrory et al.[68])

Subjects	Number of cases	GFR (ml/min/ 1.73 m² S.A.)	Serum phosphate concentration (mm/l)	Phosphate (uM/min/1.73 m² S.A.) Filtered	Resorbed	Excreted	Phosphate clearance (ml/min/ 1.73 m² S.A.)	C_{PO_4}/C_{IN}
Newborn infants (cow's milk)	5	55.5	2.34	129.0	111.0	18.0	7.7	0.14
Newborn infants (cow's milk)[a]	3	38.2	2.55	97.4	79.2	18.2	7.1	0.19
Newborn infants (human milk)[b]	9	—	1.98	—	—	6.0	3.0	—
Children[a]	6	116.6	1.65	192.4	167.0	25.4	15.4	0.13
Adults	2	133.3	1.15	153.3	144.7	8.6	7.5	0.06
Adults[c]	10	113.2	1.04	117.7	113.3	4.4	4.2	0.01
Adults[d]	4	—	1.03	—	—	13.3	12.9	—

[a] From J. B. Richmond et al.[71]
[b] From R. F. A. Dean and R. A. McCance.[72]
[c] From P. P. Lambert, E. van Kessel, and C. Leplat.[73]
[d] From R. W. Ollayos and A. W. Winkler.[74]

GFR immediately after birth limits the ability of the newborn kidney to increase phosphate excretion in response to circulating parathyroid hormone. The infants had higher GFRs on the third day, when a typical renal response was observed by these authors.

The possibility that there is a delay in onset of "adequate" parathyroid secretory activity after birth, as originally proposed by Bakwin,[67] receives additional support from the work of the Connelly group.[27] It would provide the most reasonable explanation for the well-recognized transitory hyperphosphatemia that occurs in some infants after birth. They interpreted the progressive increase in C_{PO_4}/C_{CR} ratios seen in the postnatal period as evidence of increasing secretory activity of the parathyroid gland. Other evidence in support of this view has been summarized in an excellent recent review of the subject by Anast.[69] It would appear that the major limitation imposed by renal immaturity on phosphate excretion is once more related to the GFR level. The newborn infant's quiescent parathyroid may also contribute to the development of hyperphosphatemia in the first few days under conditions of stress, since this cannot be accounted for by the relatively low level of GFR alone. The rapid postnatal rise in GFR is again seen to represent a most important maturational change which facilitates the other adjustments required postnatally in renal function as nephron size and function also increase.

Use of the Phosphate Clearance for Measurement of Renal Phosphate Excretion in Infants and Children

The actual value of the phosphate clearance is dependent on factors other than the integrity of renal function alone. Low values in growing infants may result from their active anabolic state and not from depressed renal function. The low amounts of PO_4 excreted in the urine of normal breast-fed infants, coupled with their slightly elevated levels of plasma PO_4 in comparison with normal adult plasma values, account for the low relative values of their calculated phosphate clearance. The GFR in breast-fed infants is within the same range as that of cow's-milk-fed infants who have higher values for phosphate clearance. While the finding of lower values for C_{PO_4} in breast-fed infants has been interpreted by Dean and McCance[72] as evidence of renal excretory limitation caused by immaturity of the kidney, it is more accurately interpreted as a reflection of the greater renal retention of dietary phosphate by the actively growing breast-fed newborn infant. We have shown that the ingestion of higher phosphate intakes provided by cow's milk results

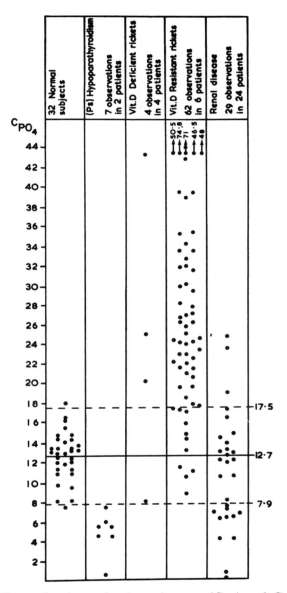

FIGURE 4.7 Twenty-four-hour phosphate clearance (C_{PO_4}) and C_{PO_4}/C_{CR} ratio in 32 normal children and in patients with abnormal phosphate metabolism. (From H. Janse, H. H. Van Gelderen, and J. H. Ruys.[76])

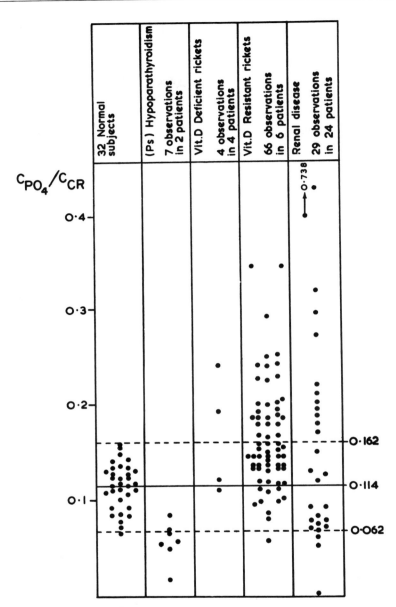

FIGURE 4.7 (continued)

in values for the newborn infants' phosphate clearance that are comparable to those in adults (Table 4.3).

The phosphate clearance is of limited value unless the state of renal function is also known. In order that the phosphate clearance can be used as an accurate measure of the integrity of renal tubular mechanisms regulating phosphate excretion, it must be related to the glomerular filtration rate, measured by either the inulin (C_{IN}) or endogenous creatinine clearance (C_{CR}), thereby giving the ratio C_{PO_4}/C_{CR}. The value of this ratio provides an estimate of the fractional rate (percent) of resorption of filtered phosphate per 100 ml of GFR.

The value of C_{PO_4}/C_{CR} provides the same information as other similar derived ratios—such as the phosphate excretion index[75] (PBI) or the percentage of filtered PO_4 resorbed[76] (TR_{PO_4})—and it seems the most direct.

The C_{PO_4}/C_{CR} ratio thus serves as the most satisfactory measure of tubular phosphate handling in normal children and subjects with abnormal phosphate metabolism (hypoparathyroidism, rickets, and vitamin D resistant rickets). While Janse, Van Gelderen, and Ruys[76] demonstrated that the 24-hour phosphate clearance (Fig. 4.7A) discriminated better than C_{PO_4}/C_{CR} (Fig. 4.7B) beween children with normal and abnormal phosphate metabolism, they recommended that the C_{PO_4}/C_{CR} ratio always be determined. It serves as a satisfactory index of tubular absorption of phosphate, at the same time providing an estimate of the GFR and thus allowing discovery of unexpected renal disease. The ratio has a further practical advantage in that it obviates errors caused by inaccurately timed urine collections.

The mean normal value of the 24-hour phosphate clearance found by these workers in children 1 to 12 years of age was 12.7 ml/min/1.73 m² S.A. with a 2 S.D. range of ± 4.8 (Fig. 4.7A). The mean value for C_{PO_4}/C_{CR} in subjects 1 to 15 years of age was 0.114 ± 0.048 (Fig. 4.7B). It was slightly higher in infants under 1 year of age. This value indicates that about 11 percent of filtered phosphate is normally being excreted.

Values for C_{PO_4} per 1.73 m² S.A. may be low in patients with markedly reduced GFR resulting from renal disease (Fig. 4.7A), but the ratio of C_{PO_4}/C_{CR} would then be normal or elevated (Fig. 4.7B). Both parameters are low in conditions associated with decreased renal excretion associated with increased tubular resorption of phosphate (hypoparathyroidism) and elevated in diseases associated with reduced rates for tubular resorption of PO_4 (hyperparathyroidism, Fanconi syndrome, and the like).

SUMMARY

The studies evaluating the quantitative capacity for physiologic renal work (water and salt excretion, acidification, and so forth) in the postnatal period have been used to document the differences that exist by quantitative comparison between newborn and older (adult) subjects in man and animals. This approach has been quite successful as an attention-getting device, but it has created an atmosphere of judgmental prejudice such that the pediatrician tends to view the newborn kidney as being functionally inadequate for the infant's needs because *it* is immature. He overlooks the fact that the newborn is also immature. As a result there has been a tendency to overemphasize and misrepresent the physiologic significance of comparative limitations that can be shown to exist in rates of renal excretion of water, solute, and electrolytes.

Our clinical experience attests to the admirable way in which the young infant's kidney regulates his water and electrolyte balance in the varied circumstances normally encountered in the postnatal period. The limits within which this renal regulatory control can respond to change and still maintain homeostasis (that is, prevent distortions in body fluid composition) have been shown to be narrowest immediately after birth; but they rapidly broaden, as evidenced by the increases in renal functional competence in the several parameters that have thus far been serially measured in the postnatal period.

There are no clinical disturbances that can be ascribed primarily to renal functional limitations in the healthy infant. When renal dysfunction does become part of a clinical problem, it usually arises as a consequence of stress of some kind and unusual or abnormal intakes either prescribed (for instance, acidified high-protein milk feedings) or associated with clinical disorders whose treatment requires some special intake, or the parenteral administration of isotonic or hypotonic electrolyte-containing fluids (such as $NaHCO_3$ infusions in the respiratory distress syndrome, parenteral alimentation with glucose and saline for neonatal sepsis or surgical management, and so forth). In this type of situation the narrow limits within which the newborn kidney can adjust to unusual requirements may be exceeded unless great precision is used in prescribing and administering special intakes in a manner appropriate to the renal functional capacity.

As mentioned in Chapter 3, renal immaturity present at birth is corrected by two mechanisms—one that is operative in the developmental maturational sense (that is, involving anatomic and cellular differentiation) and one representing adaptive growth. Both are occurring simultaneously in the neonatal period. Serial studies of certain aspects of renal function in the postnatal period have been cited that clearly show that the infant kidney possesses remarkable ability for adaptive functional growth. Our investigative curiosity should now be focused where feasible on the unique opportunity that studies of the developmental aspects of prenatal and postnatal renal function offer to define the humoral and cellular mechanisms controlling true maturational change as well as to identify the functional correlates of adaptive growth that operate pari passu postnatally but continue to operate at all ages. Such studies will probably necessitate the use of methods that will define specific functional and structural changes in renal regulation at the subcellular and single-nephron level, as well as for the total nephron aggregate making up the composite kidney.

A better understanding of the interplay between environmental stimuli and the normal processes regulating renal organ growth is of great importance to pediatrics. It seems likely that the composition and type of infant feeding is one conditioner of the rate of adaptive growth and possibly maturation of the infant's renal function. Preliminary reports have appeared from two groups[77,78] describing the effects of different dietary protein intakes on the rate of maturation of certain aspects of renal function in premature infants. Evidence of an enhanced rate of renal functional maturation has been claimed by the finding of higher values for C_{IN} and Tm_{PAH} in premature infants receiving high-protein intakes, when compared with values for these functions in comparable premature infants receiving lower-protein intakes.

Similar enhancing effects of high-protein diets could not be demonstrated in full-term infants in the studies of Calcagno and Lowe.[77] Since GFRs were not different in their subjects, the findings suggest the possibility that this effect results from stimulated maturation rather than growth hypertrophy in response to an increased work load. We cannot state at present, however, that it is desirable for all infants to be able to concentrate urine to 1,000 mOsm/l at 1 month of age, or undesirable for them to be limited in renal acid excretion in response to stress by the low-phosphate intake of breast milk. These differences in renal response do not provide a sufficient basis for preference of a particular type of diet.

It can be hoped that studies employing new techniques to correlate structure and cellular function (micropuncture studies of single nephrons and in vitro studies of the function of isolated nephron segments) will provide the information needed to gain a more complete understanding of the role of infant feeding in achieving optimal stimulation of organ growth in infancy.

From the infant's standpoint the functional ability of his kidney at birth has been shown to be quite adequate to meet his immediate needs, and his growth potential is satisfactory for future needs. The clinical implications of the finding of low values for GFR and tubular secretory capacity in newborns have been sensibly appreciated by the recommendations in the current literature that drug dosage and fluid therapy need be tailor-made to complement the now well-documented limited functional ability of the "young kidney" in the "young infant." The kidney of the newborn is not underdeveloped relative to the other parenchymal organs of the infant if viewed in the true sense of the spectrum of human developmental growth; rather, it has yet to be "stressed" by the environmental requirements unique to extrauterine life.

Chapter 5. Cellular Processes Underlying Growth and Development of the Kidney

The cellular processes responsible for development of the mature kidney involve two biologically distinct but sequential growth phases. Embryonic induction is responsible for initiating organogenesis. The second phase, postembryonic growth, is concerned with the structural and functional differentiation of the individual nephrons accounting for the unique functional traits that characterize the kidney at maturity. Embryonic growth accounts for a continuously smaller amount of cellular growth as the fetus approaches term and ceases altogether in man just before term when induction of new nephrons ceases. Although these two processes are operating simultaneously during fetal life, they should be considered as separate growth phenomena since the biochemical mechanisms regulating the two types of growth presumably involve entirely different (though possibly interacting) cellular processes.

The physiologic efficiency of the kidney depends upon the proper organization of its total number of functioning units (that is, nephrons), and this number cannot be increased after the induction of nephrons is completed. Growth of the organ after this phase will occur only by enlargement of the individual nephrons through cell division (hyperplasia) or increase in cell size (hypertrophy). The factors limiting the final structural organization of the nephrons in a manner commensurate with the requirements for efficient renal function have been discussed in Chapter 1. These principles underlie the need for allometric growth (that is to say, suitable size relations between the whole and its parts), both in embryonic and postembryonic growth.

The kidney has served as a model for many biologic investigations seeking to define the fundamental processes regulating growth of similar compound organs. The role of some of the primary biochemical regulators of embryonic growth and cell differentiation has been defined by studies employing primitive ureteric bud tissue and nephrogenic tissue (as described in Chapter 1). The cellular processes involved in renal growth by induced compensatory hypertrophy in mature mammals have also been extensively documented. Use of the kidney in the latter type of study has provided some insight into the mechanisms that presumably control the normal renal hypertrophy that accompanies growth. From observations of this type Goss[1] has constructed a conceptual framework to explain operationally how kidney size is controlled at different ages by negative feedbacks which presumably involve the same mechanisms by which its day-to-day level of functional activity is regulated.

A brief review of the current literature on cellular changes associated with renal growth is useful in order that the findings and problems of current research directed at defining the mechanisms controlling cell growth and nephron function in renal work hypertrophy can be examined for their relevance to normal renal development.

ENZYMATIC CHANGES OCCURRING WITH CELLULAR DIFFERENTIATION

The cellular changes during embryogenesis of the kidney are not yet precisely defined with respect to the specific biochemical events that initiate differentiation of nephron units except in rather general descriptive terms.

We have only fragmentary direct evidence about the subcellular events occurring with cellular differentiation which determine membrane function. The process of cellular differentiation can be considered as having been operationally initiated when the histologic criteria (both micro- and ultramicroscopic) that are diagnostic for the various specialized portions of the nephron are first identifiable. The available data make it appear probable that the potential for functional specificity, which is the end point of differentiation, may be achieved in the nephrons very shortly after their differentiation is apparent morphologically (through appearance of the glomerular basement membrane and formation of glomerular filtrate, or the presence of the brush border of the proximal convoluted tubules and active membrane transport by it).

Smith and Kissane[2] reported that morphologically recognizable glomeruli of fetal rat kidneys had essentially the same lactic dehydrogenase (LDH) activity and proportion of *A* and *B* subunits as the glomeruli of the adult kidney. Similarly the cortical proximal tubule, once it was morphologically recognizable, had the same high total LDH activity and the same high proportion of *B* subunits as the corresponding structure of the adult kidney.

Considerable presumptive evidence of a correlation between morphogenesis and the appearance of functional capability for active transport has been provided by histochemical studies showing the presence of certain enzymes (lactic dehydrogenase,[2] alkaline phosphatase,[3,4] and leucine aminopeptidase[5]) in nephrons of the fetal metanephros. The observations of Vetter and Gibley[3] and Desalu[4] show that alkaline phosphatase activity in the proximal convoluted tubules appears first at the luminal border concomitantly with development of the brush border and then appears later in intracellular loci. This sequence is compatible with lysomal activity following the onset of cell membrane transport. These observations suggest that secretory and resorptive functions are being performed by the tubules early in fetal development. Desalu did not detect either alkaline or acid phosphatase activity in undifferentiated nephrogenic tissue.

CHANGES IN RENAL ENZYME ACTIVITY AFTER BIRTH

The rapid increase in size and functional capacity of the kidney that occurs postnatally is associated with an increased rate of synthesis and activity of cellular enzymes.[6,7] The changes in gluconeogenesis occurring with renal maturation have been investigated by Zorzoli, Turkenkopf, and Mueller[7] in rat kidney in the late stages of fetal life, at birth, and during the first month of life. Adult kidney cortex tissue has been shown to have a high capacity for gluconeogenesis.[8] The Zorzoli group found that the kidney of the late fetus can synthesize glucose from either pyruvate or L-glutamate but does so at a low rate. The capacity to do so increases to levels greater than those of adult tissues during the first two postnatal weeks. These data indicate that the capacity for gluconeogenesis develops in utero in the kidney cortex and increases markedly postnatally, especially in the first two days of life. While only two enzymes were studied (glucose 6-phosphatase and phosphoenol pyruvate carboxykinase), the fact that fetal kidney cortex synthesized glucose indicates all necessary enzymes for this metabolic activity are present. The authors suggest that there is a relation between the development of significant activity of kidney phosphoenol pyruvate (PEP) in the first two days after birth and the concomitantly observed increased capacity for gluconeogenesis by kidney tissue.

The changes in the activity of some other enzymes in the postnatal period in the kidney were studied by Wacker, Zarkowsky, and Burch.[6] They measured the activity of carbonic anhydrase, glutaminase, and alkaline phosphatase from birth up to 21 days after birth and compared them with levels found in adult rats. The levels of all enzymes were low (16 to 28 percent) at birth compared to adult levels. The concentration of glutaminase and carbonic anhydrase changed very little up to 21 days; then the concentration doubled and kept increasing with age. Alkaline phosphatase levels fell postnatally but returned to levels comparable to those found at birth at 14 days and thereafter increased, tripling in value by 23 to 44 days of age. It is of interest that the 14- to 21-day period when abrupt increases in enzyme activity were noted coincides with the usual weaning period in rats and suggests that the two phenomena are associated.

As mentioned in Chapter 3, renal transport capacity for organic acids (p-aminohippurate) and bases (tetraethylammonium) is present in fetal renal cortical tissue near term in rabbits, puppies, and piglets; however, it is lower per unit of cell protein than in adult cortical tissue. The low activity persists after birth, but gradually increases to reach levels greater than that of adult tissue at 2 to 4 weeks and then declines to adult levels at 8 to 9 weeks. The observation that enzyme activity peaks at 2 to 4 weeks at levels higher than those found in adult tissue and thereafter declines to adult levels is not unique to this system; Zorzoli's group[7] found similar patterns in some of the enzymes they measured.

The rate of postnatal increase (maturation) in organic acid transport capacity (p-aminohippurate) in newborn rabbit kidney has been shown to be enhanced by the presence of substrate (penicillin) administered to the pregnant doe.[9] Even though the rate of development of increased activity was more rapid, the final level of activity did not exceed that observed in untreated animals where the peak appeared at a later time (4 weeks). This appears to be the first direct demonstration of the ability of substrate to stimulate the rate of cellular maturation of enzymatic renal tubular transport activity.

CHANGES IN RENAL NUCLEIC ACIDS AND CELL PROTEIN DURING MATURATION

An organ can increase in size either by enlarging its functional units through a greater number of cells (hyperplasia) or by increasing individual cell size (hypertrophy). During growth of any organ composed, like the kidney, of diploid cells, the cellular pattern of growth can be determined by measurements of the changes occurring in deoxyribonucleic acid (DNA), ribonucleic acid (RNA), and protein content and relating them to the weight of the organ being studied. When organ growth is occurring by hyperplasia, the increase in DNA and RNA is continuous and proportional to the weight increase and the RNA/DNA ratio remains constant. When organ growth is by cell hypertrophy, the RNA and protein content increase while DNA remains unchanged and the RNA/DNA ratio consequently increases.[10]

The cellular patterns of growth in the fetal metanephric kidney of mice late in gestation and in the postnatal period have been described by Priestley and Malt.[11] They measured the rates of cell protein and nucleic acid synthesis in fetal and postnatal and adult mice, beginning their prenatal studies at 16 days after mating of parents. They found the total protein content per cell to be low (8 percent of wet weight) 2 to 3 days before birth compared to that of the adult (16 to 17 percent of wet weight), while the fluid content is high (almost 90 percent of wet weight). Just before birth the fluid content of the kidney decreases sharply, and the protein concentration increases when related to dry weight per cell. These alterations appear to be related to physiologic changes in fetal body fluid volume compartments related to the birth process. With the exception of this perinatal change the concentration of protein continues to increase from the earliest time of study until it reaches a plateau at about 40 days of age (Fig. 5.1).

Of special interest are the changes in the RNA/DNA ratio from the earliest time of study up to maturity. The ratio decreases up to the time of birth and thereafter remains fairly constant at about 0.6 until about 20 to 30 days, when it begins to rise to achieve higher levels comparable to the adult (1.2 to 1.3 in males and 0.8 in females) at about 40 days, as shown in Fig. 5.2. The DNA content is increasing before birth and continues to rise after birth as does that of RNA during the period when the RNA/DNA ratio remains fairly constant. This would indicate that a high rate of cell division (hyperplasia) is present before birth and

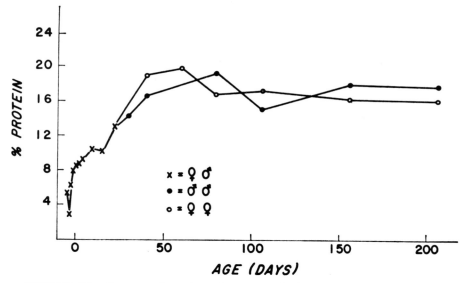

FIGURE 5.1   Concentration of total protein in mouse kidneys at different ages expressed as percentage of wet weight. (From G. C. Priestley and R. A. Malt.[11])

continues after birth until about 20 to 30 days of age before it decreases as cell hypertrophy becomes more active.

Priestley and Malt found that the concentrations of DNA and RNA reach a peak within the first week of life, after which time they both gradually decline until a relatively stable value is reached at about 40 days of age that persists with continuing growth up to 200 days. The findings of rising percentage of total cell protein mg/gm wet weight with postnatal aging and declining RNA and DNA in mg/gm dry weight are compatible with greater cytoplasmic growth (synthesis of cell protein), as might be expected with postnatal cellular functional maturation.

These changes indicate that growth by hyperplasia is most active before birth. Hyperplasia continues at a high rate until 20 to 30 days when it begins to decrease gradually; growth thereafter is increasingly a result of cell hypertrophy. The type of cell growth (hyperplasia vs hypertrophy) accounting for increasing renal size thus varies with postnatal age.

The program of cell growth in the maturing mouse kidney follows the pattern of growth in the rat described by Winick and Noble[10] for a number of organs. They have shown that growth of the rat kidney in utero and after birth to 20 to 30 days of age occurs primarily by

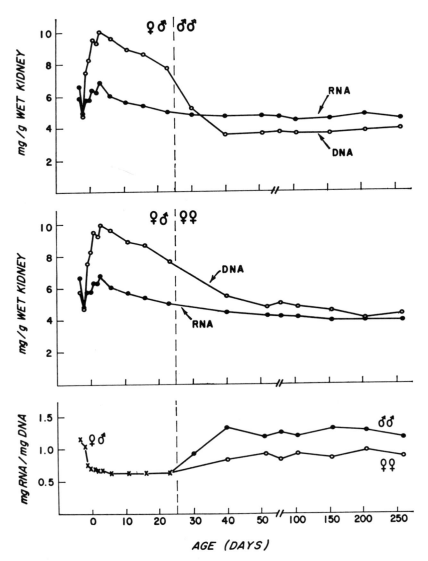

FIGURE 5.2   Concentration of nucleic acids in mouse kidneys at different ages. After 22 days of age, kidneys from males and females were analyzed separately; males are shown in the upper graph, females in the center graph, and the RNA/DNA ratios in the lower graph. (From G. C. Priestley and R. A. Malt.[11])

hyperplasia. Hyperplasia is then gradually "turned off" between 20 and 40 days, accounting for the increase in the RNA/DNA ratio. It is of interest that sexual maturation in mice occurs at about 30 days. After 40 days kidney size increases primarily by cell hypertrophy, as is evident in the stable values thereafter for the RNA/DNA ratio (see Fig. 5.2).

The mechanisms that regulate cell growth in the fetal kidney appear to be independent of those acting on cell growth of the maternal kidney. While maternal uninephrectomy in the pregnant rat has been reported[12] to stimulate growth in the fetal kidney, Goss[13] could not confirm this by finding evidence of an effect on mitotic activity of fetal kidney, and Malt and Lemaitre[14] found no change in the RNA/DNA ratio in fetal kidney even though there was clear evidence of concurrent maternal compensatory renal hypertrophy.

Striking changes in the rates of cell protein synthesis were also observed by Priestley and Malt[11] in the immediate postnatal period, suggesting that a major alteration in the "program" regulating cell protein synthesis in the fetal environment occurs at or soon after birth. The rate of protein synthesis (measured by the rate of incorporation of radioactive amino acids), which was twenty times faster in the fetal kidney than in the adult kidney, slows to twice the adult rate by 5 to 6 days after birth, even though the kidney is then entering its phase of most rapid increase in mass. The finding of a decrease in the rate of protein synthesis soon after birth is not peculiar to kidney; a similar decrease has been found in the liver[15] and the brain.[16] The experiments of Schain and his associates[16] suggest that the decrease is related to the birth event itself rather than to gestational age.

The parallel between the gradual decrease in RNA concentration in the kidney and the decrease in protein synthesis suggests that total RNA concentration may be a key factor controlling the rate of renal cell protein synthesis during growth and development. Priestley and Malt also found that most of the ribosomes isolated from fetal kidneys were free in contrast to the adult kidney where 20 to 30 percent are membrane bound. Two days after birth the proportion of bound ribosomes had risen sharply to 20 percent of the total, thereafter increasing slowly until they reached a stable level at about 30 percent of the total ribosomes in animals older than 30 days. The authors proposed that these changes may reflect the attachment of ribosomes in the early postnatal period to membranes which have been shown, by Clark's ultrastructural studies of mouse kidney,[17] to appear in quantity at this time in renal tubular cells.

INDUCED COMPENSATORY HYPERTROPHY
OF THE KIDNEY

The compensatory growth of the remaining kidney after uninephrectomy
has been used as a model for numerous studies of organ growth. These
have varied from the interest of physiologists in the nature of the changes
in renal function that permitted restoration of normal function with the
reduced renal mass to those of biologists concerned with the cellular
growth process itself. This vast subject is now covered in a book by
Nowinski and Goss[18] and will not be reviewed here in great detail. Its
relevance to the process of primary growth during normal renal development is conjectural at present because of the limited amount of direct
data. It can be assumed, however, that qualitative parallels exist between
primary adaptive growth that accounts for the continuous increase in
renal size and function that occurs from infancy up to puberty and the
secondary adaptive compensatory growth produced by uninephrectomy.
For this reason the accumulating data are of great importance to our
understanding of normal growth. The use of immature subjects is just
beginning to interest investigators working in this field. A brief summary
of the phenomena involved would seem to be of value as an orientation
to present thinking even though its applicability to developmental growth
has not been extensively explored.

Morphologic Changes

The immediate changes seen in the remaining kidney subsequent to
uninephrectomy are minimal and it takes several days to observe visible
enlargement. The initial changes reflect the increased blood flow, but
by the end of the first day actual increase in renal mass is already occurring. In the rat, for example, after 24 hours there is a true increase
in dry mass in the order of 3 percent[19] and in protein content of 18
percent.[20] The increase in dry weight is nearly linear with time in the
early postoperative period,[21] reaching 30 to 40 percent at 1 week and
about 80 percent (90 percent of the original renal mass) at predicted
equilibrium at 2 months.[22] The increments in the mouse and dog may
be slower or smaller, but the achievement at equilibrium is comparable
in restoring the renal mass of the remaining kidney nearly to the preoperative levels for two kidneys.

It is important to quantitate the normal renal growth occurring in
the sham unoperated control animals during the same observation period

as the experimental animals, or the magnitude of the stimulated growth is likely to overdramatize the actual size increase. The mass of one kidney of the normal young adult male mouse has been shown to increase 20 percent during the four-week period in which the single renoprival kidney grows 45 percent greater in mass.[22] As stated before, no new nephrons are formed during compensatory growth. The diameter of glomeruli doubles or triples.[23] Growth of the nephron involves the production of larger cells and increased numbers of cells and is most active in the proximal tubules, less active in distal tubules but still considerable, and some proliferation occurs in the ascending limbs and collecting ducts.[24,25] The increased size of the nephron is mainly a result of increased volume of glomeruli and proximal segments, the distal segments contributing little to added size.[21] Histologic evidences of tubular growth in the rat proximal tubules consist of intensified cytoplasmic basophilia which appears within hours, and soon thereafter the number of free ribosomes and small vesicles multiplies.[26] The cisternae of the rough endoplasmic reticulum dilate, the Golgi membranes and the agranular reticulum proliferate, and—by 96 hours—the number of cytoplasmic ribosomes increases further. The pattern in the distal tubules is much the same except that dedifferentiation does not seem to occur. A less differentiated type of mitotically active cell appears in the cortical portion of the collecting ducts in 72 hours.[26]

Changes in Renal Function after Uninephrectomy

In dogs following uninephrectomy, the GFR and effective renal plasma flow (ERPF) of the remaining kidney more than doubles in a day[27] and remains elevated (50 to 100 percent) for several weeks.[28] The GFR might be expected to rise almost at once, but unequivocal support of this expectation has yet to be produced in rats.[27-30] In rats of less than 250 grams, Peters[31] found that GFRs increased within two hours of occlusion of the contralateral renal pedicle and rose by 12 percent within twelve hours when effective renal plasma flow had increased 12 percent. A significant rise in GFR in rats over 250 grams does not occur until the third day, then accounting for a 65 percent restoration of the control value for two kidneys.[29]

During the first several days there is an increase in sodium excretion and urine flow, probably as a consequence of the osmotic diuresis produced by removing one kidney. Sodium resorption increases later to compensate for the alterations in sodium excretion that would otherwise result from increased GFR and ERPF. Values for Tm_{PAH} and $Tm_{GLUCOSE}$ increase one to two weeks after nephrectomy, approaching the values for both kidneys preoperatively.[27,28]

The suggestion has been made on the basis of studies with dogs that the early changes in GFR, ERPF, and water excretion result from alterations mediated by extrarenal regulatory mechanisms, while the later changes leading to altered salt and water metabolism and augmented Tm_{PAH} and $Tm_{GLUCOSE}$ are dependent on renal growth.[28]

Nephron Changes

The application of micropuncture to the study of the changes in renal sodium and water resorption in single nephrons during compensatory hypertrophy has greatly clarified how the changes come about. Since the GFR for one kidney must almost double to restore the preoperative value, tubular sodium resorption must be increased to maintain homeostasis.

The observation of Hayslett, Kashgarian, and Epstein[21] that transit time of ultrafiltrate in the proximal tubule two to four weeks after uninephrectomy in the rat is unchanged as compared with controls means that resorption in this segment does increase, for flow down the tubule is proportional to the 96 percent increase in tubular volume at this level. In the distal tubule, however, they found that transit time is lengthened 80 percent, presumably a reflection of disproportionate lengthening of Henle's loop. More transport *work* is being done in both the proximal and the distal tubules, but the distal tubules do more absorptive *work* per unit length.

Glomerulotubular balance in the nephron is maintained since the tubular fluid$_{INULIN}$/plasma$_{INULIN}$ is identical nearly everywhere in the nephron, and the rates of delivery and resorption at any point in the tubules change in proportion to the GFR. The increase in proximal tubule volume alone is therefore enough to account for a doubled resorption of filtered protein in that segment, as has been observed after uninephrectomy.[32]

Renal Functional Changes Observed with Compensatory
Growth Stimulated by Other Conditions

An increase in renal size (renal hypertrophy) associated with increases in specific functional capacity (GFR, RPF, and Tm_{PAH}) has been observed in experimental situations other than uninephrectomy. These include high intake of protein[33,34] and sodium chloride,[35] potassium deficiency,[36] chronic metabolic acidosis,[35] and parenteral injection of certain proteins such as gelatin, albumin, globulin, horseradish peroxidase, hemoglobin, and lysozyme.[37,38]

Pullman and his co-workers[34] have shown that GFR, RPF, and tubular transport capacity as measured by Tm_{PAH} show increases and decreases (± 10 percent) in normal men when they are placed on high- and low-protein intakes respectively. In an attempt to show similar effects in young infants, Calcagno and Lowe[39] found inconclusive changes in full-term infants but striking changes ($+300$ percent) in values for Tm_{PAH} in a group of premature infants receiving a protein intake of 4.8 gm of protein/kg/day, as compared to infants of similar age and weight receiving 2.2 gm of protein/kg/day. The values for GFR and RPF were not significantly different in the latter subjects, suggesting that the increase in Tm_{PAH} reflected increased cellular enzyme content. Similar results were obtained by Edelmann and Wolfish.[40] The level of dietary protein intake of the young infant thus may have an effect on the rate of maturation of certain aspects of tubular transport activity.

Adjustments in total and intrarenal blood flow are also involved in the adaptive renal functional changes found with compensatory growth. Pitts[41] has shown that the increase in GFR that occurs with high-protein feeding of dogs is brought about by changes in afferent and efferent tone whereby the effective intracapillary filtration pressure is altered. A similar mechanism could account for the increase in GFR found after high-protein intake in man,[34] in some prematures,[40] and in young and adult rats[42]; still, it seems unlikely that increases found in Tm_{PAH} in prematures by Calcagno and Lowe[39] could be accounted for by circulatory changes alone since GFR and RPF were not consistently altered.

Changes in Enzyme Activity

The fact that sodium resorption by the renal tubules increases in compensatory hypertrophy following uninephrectomy and that values for Tm_{PAH} and $Tm_{GLUCOSE}$ increase would suggest that enzyme activity is increasing per unit of membrane surface as tubular surface area increases. This has been demonstrated to occur in one instance by Katz and Epstein,[43] who found that the activity of microsomal sodium-potassium-ATPase per milligram of kidney rose 55 percent three weeks after unilateral nephrectomy as sodium resorption per milligram increased 21 percent. The importance of this change was emphasized by the absence of simultaneous increases in other microsomal enzymes (glucose 6-phosphatase, glutaminase, succinic dehydrogenase, and Mg-ATPase).

Similar changes were observed when net tubular resorption of sodium was increased by feeding high-protein diets or injection of methylprednisolone and the activity was lowered by bilateral adrenalectomy. The initiation of enzyme synthesis within tubular cells by increased contact with substrate plays a role in achieving greater functional capacity for active transport during compensatory growth. It would appear from these studies that if traffic over a pathway catalyzed by an enzyme is augmented, the amount of enzyme within the cell may increase as does the activity per milligram of cell protein. Rate-limiting enzymes have been found to be most responsive to such maneuvers.[43]

Increases in the activity of a number of other enzymes associated with proximal and distal tubules have been described following uninephrectomy. These include glutaminase,[43] glutamic dehydrogenase, and alkaline phosphatase.[44] There are also increases in glucose 6-phosphate dehydrogenase.[45] The latter are of special interest because they are the first enzymes in the hexose monophosphate shunt yielding ribose for incorporation into nucleic acids. The timing of the peak increases in their activity coincides with the peaks in mitoses of young rats.[44] The number of mitochondria in proximal tubular cells multiplies in parallel with growth of the tubules,[46] but the changes in the content of reduction-oxidation enzymes is not very marked. While succinic dehydrogenase activity is increased on the second day, cytochrome oxidase and NADH cytochrome reductase are unchanged.[47-49] Isolated normal glomeruli possess a complete complement of Krebs-cycle enzymes and neither their activity nor the ATP content changes during compensatory growth even as the glomeruli enlarge.[50]

Cellular Response in Mature Animals

Studies of the cellular growth mechanisms responsible for the increase in renal mass that follows uninephrectomy have clearly demonstrated that cell hypertrophy is the major factor contributing to the increase in organ size. Cell division is generally said to be stimulated as well,[51] although other investigators[52,53] have stated that in the rat past sexual maturation, unilateral nephrectomy stimulates compensatory hypertrophy without an increase in organ cell numbers.

Among the most detailed descriptions of the cellular phenomenon are those given by Williams[54] and Goss and Rankin.[36] Using mitotic activity as the index of cellular hyperplasia, they found that the mitotic index of cells of the proximal tubules in kidneys of mature rats did not change from the basal level of 1–2/1000 cells in the first 24 hours following uninephrectomy[55] but then rose rapidly, peaking at 40 to 48 hours and declining thereafter. Williams also found a second flurry of activity with another smaller peak between the third and fourth days. Cell division is most active in the proximal tubules.

Quantitative estimates of DNA synthesis are in accord with these morphologic signs of hyperplasia. Johnson and Vera Roman[51] measured the rate of DNA synthesis in the remaining kidney in the rat at various times for 48 hours after uninephrectomy; the pattern of change is shown in Fig. 5.3. The data were derived from counts of ^{3}H-thymidine labeling in proximal convoluted tubular epithelial cell nuclei. These authors pointed out that the choice of cells is important in interpretation of data measuring mitotic activity or cell division by change in DNA content, because the rate of DNA synthesis is greater in proximal than distal convoluted tubules. Furthermore, the variability of interstitial cell proliferation (perhaps resulting from low-grade chronic pyelonephritis) is so great in comparison with the low level of DNA synthesis in parenchymal cells that it could introduce considerable error in calculation of overall rate of DNA synthesis.

In order to clarify the sequence of cellular events, the same authors also measured rates of renal RNA and protein synthesis in the first 48 hours after nephrectomy. These data, also given in Fig. 5.3, clearly show that after nephrectomy the initial response of the remaining kidney is increased RNA synthesis within the first hour, followed some 18 hours later by a rise in DNA synthesis which reaches a maximum at 48 hours. To compare the effects of hyperplasia and hypertrophy, they calculated the contribution that the increase in cell population could be assigned in accounting for the increase in dry weight. By the end of the fifth day, when DNA synthesis has passed its peak, cellular hyperplasia accounts for only one-fourth of the observed increase in kidney weight (see Fig. 5.4). The increase in weight of the renoprival kidney is thus largely accounted for by increased cell protein synthesis rather than by new cell formation.

The types of cell proteins formed have been identified by Malt and Miller,[56] who measured the sequential changes in classes of RNA during compensatory growth of the kidney in young (42- to 50-day-old) adult mice. The amount of RNA in the average cell begins to increase soon

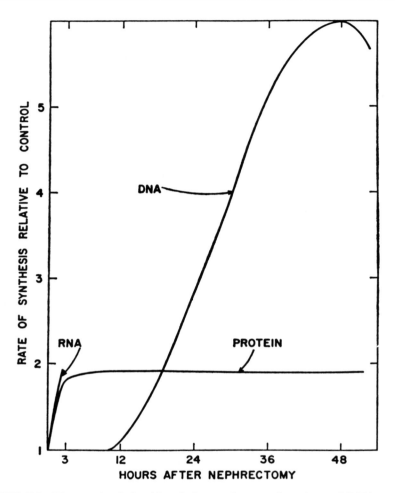

FIGURE 5.3   Temporal relationship of changes in rate of synthesis of RNA, protein, and DNA in remaining kidney after uninephrectomy. (From H. A. Johnson and J. M. Vera Roman.[51])

after contralateral nephrectomy and approaches its maximum two to four days later. During this time there is a two- to fourfold increase in the rate of formation of ribosomes, and more polyribosomes are recoverable from equivalent masses of renal tissue. Malt and Miller interpreted their findings as indicating that the initial increase in RNA in the renoprival state appears to be caused by enhanced synthesis of the nuclear precursors of ribosomal RNA (*rnuc* RNA). The peaks in the amounts of *rnuc* RNA formed (steadily increasing until the second day and then falling to rise again on the eighth day) coincide nicely with the waves of mitotic activity in mice and rats.[51,54,57] The changes in messenger RNA (*m* RNA) are quite the reverse: this substance is present in low amounts on the second day after nephrectomy, when *rnuc* RNA is high.

The authors cite the similarities between their findings and those of other workers who employed rabbit kidney fragments stimulated to grow in tissue culture[58] and rat spleen and lymph nodes stimulated to produce antibody by immunization.[59] Predominant synthesis of *rnuc* RNA has been found to be a characteristic of the dividing cell, whereas *m* RNA accumulates in the nondividing cell.[60]

The degree of cellular hypertrophy and/or hyperplasia that occurs following unilateral nephrectomy is affected by important extrarenal factors that also influence growth. These include protein and caloric intake,

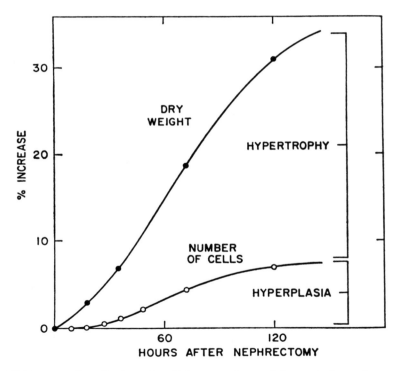

FIGURE 5.4 Contribution of cell hypertrophy and hyperplasia to increase in mass in dry weight after uninephrectomy in mature rat. (From H. A. Johnson and J. M. Vera Roman.[51])

since high-protein feeding stimulates[61] and starvation suppresses compensatory hypertrophy and hyperplasia even in weanling rats.[62] In addition, hormonal factors (pituitary, sex, and adrenal), presence or absence of infection, and trauma influence the response. The effects of these factors are extensively dealt with elsewhere[1,63] and will not be considered in detail here.

CHEMICAL CONTROL OF CELLULAR GROWTH IN RENAL COMPENSATORY HYPERTROPHY

The description in biochemical terms of the sequence of cellular events following uninephrectomy provides a basis for defining the "program" that regulates renal hypertrophy. The initial step appears to be an increase in RNA and cell protein synthesis. Since DNA synthesis is a prerequisite of mitosis, one would expect the onset of DNA synthesis to parallel that of increased mitotic activity and precede it by some reasonable time interval. There are data to support this expectation.[51,63]

The initial RNA response that occurs has been proposed as the first cellular response to increased functional load (that is, simple "work hypertrophy"). The interval between these changes and the onset of DNA synthesis was interpreted by Johnson and Vera Roman as suggesting that factors which control compensatory growth of the kidney, whatever they may be, do not act primarily by regulation of DNA synthesis but by regulation of RNA and protein synthesis. This implies a corollary "that in this case cell proliferation occurs secondary to cell hypertrophy, that a cell divides only if and when it reaches a certain critical size or perhaps a certain critical ratio of cytoplasm to nucleus."[51]

The possibility also arises that proliferation follows hypertrophy in response to an unsatisfied need for augmented renal functional capacity. The data of Malt and Miller[56] support the hypothesis that the stimulus (or stimuli) to compensatory hypertrophy may operate by initiating ribosomal RNA synthesis either directly or by depletion of cellular stores of messenger RNA, and that production of the latter could be triggered by the early increase in ribosomal RNA or by a precipitous decrement in ribosomal RNA. If this is the case, the stimulus to compensatory hypertrophy need operate for only a short time to set in motion a complex series of events that can be responsible for cellular hypertrophy—or if cell size is regulated by optimal cytoplasmic nuclear ratios, to initiate cell division when these are exceeded. The proposal also assumes that there may be a common cause, whether mediated by changes in functional load (work hypertrophy) or loss of renal mass that triggers release of a substance that sets the sequence for hypertrophy and potentially hyperplasia in motion.

Malt considers the simple work hypothesis unlikely,[63] but this stems more from the present confusion because of the lack of agreement on how to quantify renal work than from unequivocal evidence providing direct answers to the alternatives raised. He does point out the absence of proof that new species or quantities of RNA are required for synthesis of new transport enzymes or other cytoplasmic proteins. The hypotheses of a common pathway are of value because they may confine the search for the cause of compensatory growth. The relevance of these studies to the processes regulating normal renal growth in the newborn and young subject is still conjectural since few pertinent data are available.

EFFECTS OF AGE ON CELLULAR RESPONSE TO UNINEPHRECTOMY

The pattern of cellular growth in the kidney changes in the postnatal period as described earlier. The rate of cell hyperplasia is highest in the newborn of all species and accounts for most of the increase in organ size that takes place. The contribution of hyperplasia to postnatal organ growth decreases as age increases.[10] It is known that mitotic activity is greatest in the kidney at birth and least in old age.[64] It has also been demonstrated that the degree of compensatory hypertrophy observed after uninephrectomy decreases with advancing age.[65] Phillips and Leong[64] found that hyperplasia accounts for a greater portion of the increase in weight of a renoprival kidney in a young rat than in a mature rat. They found that the cellular response in the 30-day-old weanling rat, while qualitatively similar to that of a 4-month-old adult rat (peak DNA synthesis at 36 hours), demonstrated more proliferative activity as judged by changes in the mitotic index.

The weanling rat is not comparable to the human "weanling" because the period of time required for the rat to begin maturing sexually is quite short (about 30 days) and cell growth after sexual maturation is predominantly by cell hypertrophy.[52,53] Investigators have been forced to use weanling rats (then 20 to 30 days of age) because of their inability to artificially feed the newborn rat successfully during the normal weanling period. There are little data, consequently, on the response of the newborn rat to nephrectomy.

The development of an efficient technique for artificial feeding allowed

Karp, Brasel, and Winick[66] to examine the response of the 4-day-old infant rat to uninephrectomy and compare it with that of 40-day-old and 3- to 4-month-old rats. They demonstrated the quantitative cellular changes that are seen in the response of the renoprival kidney when growth by hyperplasia is normally most active. The initial sequence of cellular events following uninephrectomy in the 4-day-old infant rat is identical to the adult. At 12 hours there is a rise in protein content and in protein/DNA ratio, and by 24 hours the RNA content also has increased. These changes are indicated in Table 5.1. Unlike the adult, however, the DNA content of the renoprival kidney in the young animal is also significantly elevated at 24 hours. Autoradiography shows that there is increased uptake of DNA precursors in both glomerular and tubular cells. By 7 days there is a 22 percent increase in DNA in comparison to the sham kidney, without an increase in protein/DNA ratio or change in RNA/DNA ratio; this implies that hyperplasia has occurred without hypertrophy. By 14 days, however, there is evidence of some hypertrophy (increase in protein/DNA ratio), and by about 40 days hypertrophy has become predominant as evidenced by the increase in protein/DNA and RNA/DNA ratios.

The normal cellular growth pattern in rat kidney at 40 days of age and after is one of growth by hypertrophy.[10] The changes in nucleic acid content and protein vary with age when the values in the renoprival kidney and sham kidney are compared two weeks after nephrectomy. Table 5.2 gives the results of Karp, Brasel, and Winick[66] for 40-day-old and 3- to 4-month-old rats, which can be compared with those observed at 14 days following uninephrectomy in the 4-day-old rat (Table 5.1). The 3- to 4-month-old rat responded with cell hypertrophy, since the DNA content was similar to that of the sham animal's kidney; furthermore, the protein/DNA and RNA/DNA ratios increased, indicating cell hypertrophy had occurred.

The type of cellular response to uninephrectomy is thus an age-dependent phenomenon and the degree of hyperplasia or hypertrophy observed postoperatively will depend on the subject's age at the time of sampling. The 4-day-old infant rat's response to uninephrectomy represents an augmented pattern of hyperplasia, which is the existing growth pattern as can be seen in the animal that had the sham operation. As stated above, in the postpubertal rat unilateral nephrectomy stimulates an increase in weight, protein, and RNA in the remaining kidney without an increase in the number of cells in the organ when compared to con-

TABLE 5.1 Changes in weight, protein, RNA, and DNA content of the remaining total kidney following uninephrectomy in 4-day-old rats (from R. Karp, J. A. Brasel, and M. Winick[66])

Time post-operative	No. of animals studied[a]	Weight (mg)	Protein[b] (mg)	DNA[b] (mg)	Protein/DNA[b]	RNA (mg)	RNA/DNA
12 hours	R6	72	4.9(0.025)	0.51(NS)	9.65(<0.001)	0.49(NS)	0.96
	S7	73	3.8	0.55	8.12	0.47	0.86
24 hours	R10	84	4.8(NS)	0.52(<0.001)	9.22(NS)	0.51(<0.001)	0.98
	S8	75	4.3	0.47	9.10	0.45	0.96
3 days	R4	98	8.6(0.05)	0.62(0.025)	13.9(NS)	0.64(<0.001)	1.03
	S5	87	7.4	0.56	13.0	0.52	0.92
7 days	R4	160	15.6(0.01)	0.94(<0.001)	16.7(NS)	0.84(<0.001)	0.90
	S5	126	11.6	0.77	15.0	0.68	0.88
14 days	R3	317	33.0(<0.001)	1.71(<0.001)	19.3(0.01)	1.64(<0.001)	0.96
	S5	218	24.6	1.38	17.9	1.25	0.91
41 days	R8	1,345	172.7(<0.001)	3.24(<0.001)	54.0(<0.001)	4.40(<0.001)	1.36
	S6	774	87.1	2.83	30.7	3.30	1.16

[a] R = renoprival; S = sham.
[b] (0.025) = p values; NS = not significant.

TABLE 5.2 Changes in weight, protein, RNA, and DNA content of the remaining total kidney two weeks after uninephrectomy in 40-day-old and 3- to 4-month-old rats (from R. Karp, J. A. Brasel, and M. Winick[66])

Kidney	40-day-old rats		3- to 4-month-old male rats	
	Renoprival[a]	Sham	Renoprival[a]	Sham
Time postoperative	14 days	14 days	13 days	13 days
No. of animals	3	2	10	10
Weight (gm)	1.15	0.94	1.84	1.45
Protein (mg)	166.6 (<0.001)	120.9	445 (<0.001)	309
DNA (mg)	4.39 (0.01)	3.10	4.26 (NS)	4.00
Protein/DNA	38.5 (NS)	38.7	107 (0.01)	78
RNA (mg)	5.86	4.21	6.35 (<0.001)	4.98
RNA/DNA	1.36	1.43	1.50	1.25

[a] (0.001) = p values; NS = not significant.

trols.[52,53] The data of the Karp group support this conclusion. The cellular response may, however, be influenced by other factors as well; McCreight and Sulkin[55] reported that the deletion of progressively larger portions of renal tissue (up to seven-eighths total nephrectomy) led to increased mitotic activity in the renoprival proximal convoluted tubule.

This age-dependent difference in response is similar to that found by Winick and Noble for other organs. These researchers have shown that an organ's growth response when experimentally altered differs depending on the age of the subject and the nature of the existing pattern of cell growth.[10,67] When growth in a particular organ is occurring primarily by hyperplasia, a growth stimulus augments it still further. This would explain why the response to the same experimental situation differs in the sexually mature rat, where stimulated renal growth takes place primarily by cell hypertrophy. The cellular mechanisms responsible for these age-related differences have not been identified. Studies aimed at clarifying them will require that the age of the animals selected be chosen in a most careful manner especially when dealing with rapidly maturing animals.

THE ROLE OF INCREASED RENAL WORK LOAD IN STIMULATING RENAL GROWTH

The increase in size of the remaining kidney after uninephrectomy has usually been viewed operationally as work hypertrophy, but the identity of the stimulus is controversial. Uninephrectomy decreases the complement of nephrons (renal mass) as well as increasing the work load for the remaining renal mass. Numerous experimental studies have been designed to separate the effects of increased renal excretory load from the effects of a reduction in renal cell mass. The procedures have been complicated and the results conflicting.

Attempts to separate these two factors have included (1) ligation or transsection of one ureter without removal of renal tissue; and (2) diversion of urine output from one kidney by transplantation of its ureter to the gut or peritoneal cavity, thus increasing the functional load to both kidneys without reducing renal mass. Ligation of one ureter has proved to be a stimulus to compensatory hypertrophy (involving hyperplasia) of the nonobstructed kidney.[36,68,69] Benitez and Shaka[69] found that the cortex of the kidney on the obstructed side showed greater mitotic activity (measured by mitotic counts and ^{3}H-thymidine uptake) than did the cortex of the unobstructed contralateral kidney. This suggests that distention secondary to increased intrapelvic pressure may also stimulate renal hyperplasia; however, other explanations (such as infection or reaction to trauma) are equally plausible.

Simpson[70] reported that increasing renal excretory load without reducing renal mass did not result in hyperplasia. He attempted to achieve this by diversion of urine output of one kidney into the peritoneal cavity by ureteral transplantation. Royce,[71] however, later performed similar studies and found that trauma associated with peritoneostomy and the resulting postoperative food and water restriction, as well as induction of peritonitis by talc instillation, eliminated the proliferative renal response typically seen after uncomplicated unilateral nephrectomy. Phillips and Wachtel[62] confirmed Royce's findings. Eckert, Kountz, and Cohn[72] subsequently reported that diversion of the ureter without the obstructive or infectious complications mentioned above reduces but does not prevent some compensatory renal hypertrophy involving both kidneys. The importance of these two factors (work load and total functioning renal mass) in regulating renal function is thus difficult to assess and is still under study.

A role for humoral factors has been suggested by reports that serum ribonuclease activity rises after bilateral nephrectomy[73] and that serum from unilaterally nephrectomized rats stimulates hyperplasia in normal kidney cells in vitro.[74] Rabinovitch and Dohi[73] attributed the rise in serum ribonuclease concentration to its reduced renal clearance. Royce[38] has demonstrated that renal weight gain in the rat produced by the injection of egg white lysozyme (a small 17,500 molecular weight protein filtered by the glomerulus and resorbed by the proximal tubule) is associated with increased synthesis of DNA in the epithelial cells of the renal tubule. He has shown that serum ribonuclease is handled by the renal tubular cell in a manner similar to lysozyme, horseradish peroxidase, and hemoglobin. Both the plasma concentration and renal uptake of plasma ribonuclease are increased by unilateral nephrectomy. Royce suggests that alterations in rate of renal resorption and degradation of serum ribonuclease and other filtrate proteins may play a role in elevating serum levels and in mediating compensatory renal hyperplasia. With any decrease in renal functional mass there would be an increase in serum level because of decreased renal removal.

Kurnick and Lindsay,[75] in studies using parabiotic mice, have reported that a stimulus to renal hypertrophy can be transmitted humorally. The nature of the stimulus is not known, however, and the evidence on which its existence is postulated has been questioned.[63] The existence of a transferable serum factor, postulated by Lowenstein and Stern[74] as being capable of stimulating mitotic activity in the kidneys of normal rats, has also been questioned since Kurnick and Lindsay[75] and Williams[54] were unable to confirm these observations. The role of humoral mediation of changes resulting from an increase in renal work load is still uncertain. The studies of Eckert, Kountz, and Cohn[72] have suggested that humoral mediation may be less effective than a significant decrease in total renal mass, but the possibility cannot be ignored that either may produce a humoral stimulus initiating hypertrophy.

WHAT IS THE RENAL WORK LOAD?

A major difficulty in resolving this controversy arises from the lack of agreement in the literature as to how one defines renal work load. The concept that the kidney performs work in the elaboration of urine is as rational as is the unavoidable conclusion that this work must be increased for the remaining kidney after uninephrectomy. It is obvious that more blood is available for processing by the remaining kidney. The actual increase in renal work load associated with the increase in perfusion cannot be quantitated, however, until some generally acceptable definition of renal excretory work is provided.

A very provocative and stimulating discussion of this problem has been presented by Johnson and Knudsen.[76] The excretion of urine with its contained electrolytes and metabolites has long been considered the major work performed by the kidney. From this standpoint the definition of renal work is dependent on the differences that can be demonstrated between the composition of an ultrafiltrate of plasma and the final urine, in terms of osmotic concentration achieved, urea excreted, and so forth. Such a definition is quite unsatisfactory because the excretion of urine in this sense would use only a fraction of 1 percent of the energy supplied to the kidney under normal conditions, leaving a large energy reserve.

The kidney is the primary regulator of the volume and composition of body fluids and its excretory function is incidental to its regulatory function. Johnson and Knudsen point out that tubular resorption of glomerular filtrate represents most of the functional load, and consideration of the work load involved in electrolyte resorption leads to the conclusion that the kidney works quite efficiently with a small margin of unused energy. They apply communication-theory systems of analysis to simulate the problems faced by the kidney in its work role—such as identification of those selected ions (sodium, for example) that must be almost completely resorbed from filtrate. The discrimination in selection of individual ions like sodium from all other constituents of glomerular filtrate requires work if it is to be responsive to feedback controls, but most work is accounted for by the energy utilized in ion resorption which involves active membrane and transcellular ion transport. These authors present theoretic data to show that the energy consumed by the kidney can be largely accounted for by "work" performed to meet the daily requirements of resorption of 98 percent or more of the filtered load of sodium and other major ions. By these calculations the kidney can be shown to operate with a high level of efficiency (40 percent) for work done per energy consumed.

The approach is attractive because it proposes that renal work be quantitated in terms that allow the processes involved (such as sodium resorption) to be directly measured experimentally. At the present time there is no agreement on the bases that will best define renal work load in quantitative terms. Since quantitative tubular resorption of filtered sodium represents the greatest part of the functional load of the kidney, it would be most sensitive to major changes in glomerular filtration; measurements of the rate of tubular resorption should therefore reflect changes in overall energy expenditure. In view of these observations, experiments designed to test the "functional load" hypothesis should demonstrate a change in overall tubular sodium resorption if there is to be direct evidence to document a presumed increase in functional load. The value of this approach is evident in the elegant observations by Katz and Epstein[43] measuring changes in sodium-potassium-ATPase and sodium resorption following uninephrectomy in the rat.

SUMMARY

It appears probable that functional specificity (the end point of differentiation) is achieved by cells comprising the nephrons during fetal morphogenesis, concomitantly with the appearance of histologic criteria that characterize the various portions of the nephrons. The data that support this view come from correlative studies comparing enzymatic activity with morphologic evidence of differentiation. The measurements of changes in enzyme activity in the postnatal period have documented increases in the activity of enzymes involved in gluconeogenesis and in activity of carbonic anhydrase, glutaminase, and alkaline phosphatase. The pattern of change is one of a slow rise in enzymatic activity up to 14 to 21 days after birth when changes occur with a peak achieved after weaning, following which the activity falls to levels comparable to those of adult kidney tissue. The increase observed in enzymatic activity of renal proximal tubular cells correlates well with the functional evidence that transport capacity of the proximal tubules is increasing simultaneously.

The cellular pattern of fetal growth is predominantly one of growth by hyperplasia. The rate of protein synthesis (in vitro) of subcellular ribosomes from fetal kidney tubules is greater than that in postnatal renal tissue, even though growth by hyperplasia is very active postnatally—at least for the first 20 days in the rat. The ribosomes are not membrane bound to any great extent in the fetal kidney cells but become so in increasing amounts in the first two days after birth. This may reflect their attachment to membranes which begin to appear in quantity at this time. The cellular pattern of kidney growth changes from the hyperplasia characteristic of the first 20 days to one of predominant hypertrophy by 40 to 50 days, an event that coincides with sexual maturity.

The cellular response of the kidney to the growth stimulus of uninephrectomy varies with age. The young infant responds with augmented hyperplasia, while the sexually mature rat responds primarily by enlargement via cell hypertrophy. The stimulus to renal compensatory hypertrophy has not been identified but is attributed to increased requirements for "renal work"—even though what comprises "renal work" has not been clearly defined in quantitative physiologic terms. The humoral and subcellular regulators of cell hyperplasia and/or hypertrophy have yet to be defined, but the sequence begins with increased RNA and cell protein synthesis. The stimulus to cell division has been postulated to arise when the work load stimulus is in excess of the augmentation achieved by the compensatory response of cell hypertrophy alone.

The relevance of the functional-morphologic correlates of renal compensatory hypertrophy to normal renal growth during maturation is conjectural at present. The data are of great interest, nonetheless, because the processes involved are probably qualitatively similar. This is indicated by the comparable immediate changes in cellular nucleic acid and protein synthesis in the infant and adult rat following uninephrectomy. The mechanisms regulating the quantitative age-dependent differences in this response have not yet been defined.

The "work load" hypothesis as a cause of renal compensatory hypertrophy when applied to infants has obvious special implications for infant feeding. The protein content of normal feedings of infants may represent, in part, an important stimulus to enzymatic synthesis via substrate induction. The predominant type of cellular growth pattern in the infant (hyperplasia) may also be a conditioning factor, although this is speculation. The exogenous work load presented by the dietary intake would serve as an additional stimulus to the augmentation of the endogenous renal regulatory work load that results from continuously increasing body mass and fluid volumes (cellular and extracellular) during the rapid growth observed in the mammal postnatally.

We do not yet know which factors trigger normal renal maturation, or whether they involve the same mechanisms that regulate adult renal growth. The functional correlates (glomerulotubular balance) may be quantitatively different, since the cellular patterns of growth differ in the newborn from those characteristic of sexually mature animals. A more complete description of the duration and controls responsible for the normal period of growth by cellular maturation, hypertrophy, and hyperplasia is required before it will be possible to determine whether inhibition during the phase of active growth in the prenatal and postnatal period can have any long-lasting effect on the functional work potential of the kidney in adult life.

Notes and Index

Notes

CHAPTER 1. EMBRYOLOGIC DEVELOPMENT OF THE KIDNEY

1. J. Oliver, *Nephrons and Kidneys: A Quantitative Study of Developmental and Evolutionary Mammalian Renal Architectonics* (New York: Hoeber Medical Division, Harper and Row, 1968), p. 43.

2. R. J. Goss, *Adaptive Growth* (London: Logos Press Ltd., 1964).

3. J. Oliver, When is the kidney not a kidney? (Ramon Guiteras Memorial Lecture), *J Urol* 63:373, 1950.

4. R. Platt, M. H. Roscoe, and F. W. Smith, Experimental renal failure, *Clin Sci* 11:217, 1952.

5. A. B. Morrison, Experimentally induced chronic renal insufficiency in the rat, *Lab Invest* 11:321, 1962.

6. R. Platt, Structural and functional adaptation in renal failure (Lumleian Lecture), *Brit Med J* 1:1313, 1952.

7. N. S. Bricker, S. Klahr, H. Lubowitz, and R. E. Rieselbach, Renal function in chronic renal disease, *Medicine (Balt)* 44:263, 1965.

8. J. M. Kissane, Congenital malformations, in *Pathology of the Kidney*, ed. R. H. Heptinstall (Boston: Little, Brown and Company, 1966), chap. 3.

9. J. Bernstein, Developmental abnormalities of the renal parenchyma—renal hypoplasia and dysplasia, in *Pathology Annual 1968,* ed. S. C. Sommers (New York: Appleton-Century-Crofts [Meredith Corporation], 1968), vol. 3, p. 213.

10. Oliver, note 1, p. 58.

11. A. Ljungqvist and C. Lagergren, The Ask-Upmark kidney. A congenital renal anomaly studied by micro-angiography and histology, *Acta Path Microbiol Scand* 56:277, 1962.

12. P. Royer, R. Habib, V. Courtecuisse, and F. Leclerc, L'hypoplasie rénale bilatérale avec oligonéphronie (étude de 21 observations), *Arch Franç Pédiat* 24:249, 1967.

13. R. F. Pitts, *Physiology of the Kidney and Body Fluids,* ed. 2 (Chicago: Year Book Medical Publishers, Inc., 1968), pp. 17–18.

14. K. Peter, *Untersuchungen über Bau und Entwicklung der Niere* (Jena: Gustav Fischer Verlag, 1909).

15. W. Felix, The development of the urogenital organs, in *Manual of Human Embryology,* ed. F. Keibel and F. P. Mall (Philadelphia: J. B. Lippincott, 1910–1912), vol. 2.

16. C. M. Bennett, B. M. Brenner, and R. W. Berliner, Micropuncture study of nephron function in the rhesus monkey, *J Clin Invest* 47:203, 1968.

17. Pitts, note 13, pp. 18 and 118.

18. K. Thurau, Renal hemodynamics, *Amer J Med* 36:698, 1964.

19. M. Horster and K. Thurau, Micropuncture studies on the filtration rate of single superficial and juxtamedullary glomeruli in the rat kidney, *Pflueger Arch Ges Physiol* 301:162, 1968.

20. B. H. Pomeranz, A. G. Birtch, and A. C. Barger, Neural control of intrarenal blood flow, *Amer J Physiol* 215:1067, 1968.

21. L. B. Arey, *Developmental Anatomy: A Textbook and Laboratory Manual of Embryology,* ed. 6 (Philadelphia: W. B. Saunders & Co., 1954).

22. B. M. Patten, *Human Embryology,* ed. 3 (New York: McGraw-Hill Book Company, 1968), pp. 450–451.

23. A. M. Du Bois, The embryonic kidney, in *The Kidney: Morphology, Biochemistry, Physiology,* ed. C. Rouiller and A. F. Muller (New York: Academic Press, 1969), vol. 1, chap. 1.

24. T. W. Torrey, The early development of the human nephros, *Contrib Embryol* (no. 231–241) 35:175, 1954.

25. M. R. Vetter and C. W. Gibley, Jr., Morphogenesis and histochemistry of the developing mouse kidney, *J Morph* 120:135, 1966.

26. E. A. Fraser, The development of the vertebrate excretory system, *Biol Rev* 25:159, 1950.

27. Athanasian Creed, in *The Book of Common Prayer of The Church of England* (London: Oxford University Press, 1899), p. 56.

28. J. M. Kissane, Development of the kidney, in *Pathology of the Kidney,* ed. R. H. Heptinstall (Boston: Little, Brown and Company, 1966), chap. 2.

29. D. I. Williams, The foetal ureter, *Brit J Urol* 23:366, 1951.

30. R. Chwalle, The process of formation of cystic dilatations of the vesical end of the ureter and of diverticula at the ureteral ostium, *Urol Cutan Rev* 31:499, 1927.

31. L. Gyllensten, Contributions to the embryology of the human bladder; development of definitive relations between openings of Wolffian ducts and ureters, *Acta Anat* 7:305, 1949.

32. I. Gersh, The correlation of structure and function in the developing mesonephros and metanephros, *Contrib Embryol* (no. 153) 26:35, 1937.

33. A. Giroud, Causes and morphogenesis of anencephaly, in *Ciba Foundation Symposium on Congenital Malformations,* ed. G. E. W. Wolstenholme and C. M. O'Connor (Boston: Little, Brown and Company, 1960), p. 199.

34. H. Spemann, *Embryonic Development and Induction* (New Haven, Conn.: Yale University Press, 1938).

35. C. Grobstein, Inductive interaction in the development of the mouse metanephros, *J Exp Zool* 130:319, 1955.

36. E. Wolff, E. Wolff, and S. Bishop-Calame, Explants of embryonic tissue: techniques and applications, in *The Kidney: Morphology, Biochemistry, Physiology,* ed. C. Rouiller and A. F. Muller (New York: Academic Press, 1969), vol. 2, chap. 1.

37. C. Grobstein, Some transmission characteristics of the tubule-inducing influence on mouse metanephrogenic mesenchyme, *Exp Cell Res* 13:575, 1957.

38. E. Zwilling, Interaction between limb bud ectoderm and mesoderm in the chick embryo. II. Experimental limb duplications, *J Exp Zool* 132:173, 1956.

39. J. D. Ebert, The acquisition of biological specificity, in *The Cell: Biochemistry, Physiology, Morphology,* ed. J. Brachet and A. E. Mirsky (New York: Academic Press, 1959), vol. 1, p. 619.

40. M. Winick and R. E. Greenberg, Chemical control of sensory ganglia during a critical period of development, *Nature (London)* 205:180, 1965.

41. M. Winick and W. W. McCrory, Renal differentiation: a model for the study of development, in *Birth Defects: Original Article Series,* ed. D. Bergsma (New York: National Foundation, 1968), vol. 4, no. 5.

42. E. D. Hay, Recent studies of embryonic induction, *New Eng J Med* 268:1114, 1963.

43. Oliver, note 1, p. 3.

44. W. Bowman, On the structure and use of the Malpighian bodies of the kidney, with observations on circulation through that gland, *Philos. Tr. Roy. Soc. London* 132:57, 1842.

45. P. T. Herring, The development of the Malpighian bodies of the kidney, and its relation to pathological changes which occur in them, *J Path Bact* 6:459, 1900.

46. K. W. Zimmerman, Über den Bau des Glomerulus der Säugerniere. Weitere Mitteilungen, *Z Mikr Anat Forsch* 32:176, 1933.

47. W. von Möllendorff, Über Deckzellen und Bindegewebe im Glomerulus der menschlichen Niere, *Z Zellforsch* 11:46, 1930.

48. S. M. Kurtz and J. F. A. McManus, A reconsideration of the development, structure, and disease of the human renal glomerulus, *Amer Heart J* 58:357, 1959.

49. B. V. Hall, Further studies of the normal structure of the renal glomerulus, in *Proceedings of the Sixth Annual Conference on the Nephrotic Syndrome, 1954* (New York: National Nephrosis Foundation, Inc., 1955).

50. S. M. Kurtz, The electron microscopy of the developing human renal glomerulus, *Exp Cell Res* 14:355, 1958.

51. Oliver, note 1, p. 10.

52. O. J. Lewis, The development of the blood vessels of the metanephros, *J Anat* 92:84, 1958.

53. A. Aoki, Development of the human renal glomerulus. I. Differentiation of the filtering membrane, *Anat Rec* 155:339, 1966.

54. Y. Suzuki, An electron-microscopical study of renal differentiation. II. The glomerulus, *Keio J Med* 8:129, 1959.

55. J. Davies, *Human Developmental Anatomy* (New York: Ronald Press, 1963).

56. V. Osathanondh and E. L. Potter, Development of human kidney as shown by microdissection. V. Development of vascular pattern of glomerulus, *Arch Path (Chicago)* 82:403, 1966.

57. B. F. Trump and R. E. Bulger, Morphology of the kidney, in *Structural Basis of Renal Disease,* ed. E. L. Becker (New York: Hoeber Medical Division, Harper and Row, 1968), chap. 1.

58. R. E. Coupland, The anatomy of the human kidney, in *Renal Disease,* ed. 2, ed. D. A. K. Black (Oxford: Blackwell Scientific Publications, 1967), chap. 1.

59. A. Maximow, Tissue-cultures of young mammalian embryos, *Contrib Embryol* (no. 80) 16:47, 1925.

60. P. Gruenwald, Stimulation of nephrogenic tissue by normal and abnormal inductors, *Anat Rec* 86:321, 1943.

61. R. L. Vernier and A. Birch-Andersen, Studies of the human fetal kidney. I. Development of the glomerulus. *J Pediat* 60:754, 1962.

62. C. B. McLoughlin, Mesenchymal influences on epithelial differentiation, in *Cell Differentiation,* Symposia of the Society for Experimental Biology (New York: Academic Press, 1963), no. 17, p. 359.

63. P. M. Bloom, J. F. Hartmann, and R. L. Vernier, An electron microscopic evaluation of the width of normal glomerular basement membrane in man at various ages (abst.), *Anat Rec* 133:251, 1959.

64. O. F. Kampmeier, A hitherto unrecognized mode of origin of congenital renal cysts, *Surg Gynec Obstet* 36:208, 1923.

65. Oliver, note 1, p. 5.

66. G. C. Huber, On the development and shape of uriniferous tubules of certain of the higher mammals, *Amer J Anat,* vol. 4, suppl. 1, 1905.

67. A. Ljungqvist, Fetal and postnatal development of the intrarenal arterial pattern in man. A micro-angiographic and histologic study, *Acta Paediat* 52:443, 1963.

68. G. Cameron and R. Chambers, Direct evidence of function in kidney of an early human fetus, *Amer J Physiol* 123:482, 1938.

69. Oliver, note 1, p. 36.

70. Ibid., p. 37.

71. E. Moberg, Anzahl und Grösse der Glomeruli renales beim Menschen nebst Methoden, diese zahlenmässig festzustellen, *Z Mikr Anat Forsch* 18:271, 1929.

72. E. L. Potter and S. Thierstein, Glomerular development in the kidney as an index of fetal maturity, *J Pediat* 22:695, 1943.

73. M. S. Macdonald and J. L. Emery, The late intrauterine and postnatal development of human renal glomeruli, *J Anat* 93:331, 1959.

74. E. D. Korn, Current concepts of membrane structure and function, *Fed Proc* 28:6, 1969.

75. R. K. Crane, A concept of the digestive-absorptive surface of the small intestine, in *Handbook of Physiology,* ed. C. F. Code (Washington, D.C.: American Physiological Society, 1968), vol. 5, sec. 6, *Alimentary Canal.*

76. R. L. Vernier and F. G. Smith, Jr., Fetal and neonatal kidney, in *Biology of Gestation,* ed. N. S. Assali (New York: Academic Press, 1968), vol. 2, chap. 5.

77. C. W. Gibley, The histochemistry of the developing pro- and mesonephros of the chick embryo (abst.), *Amer Zool* 4:402, 1964.

78. D. P. Alexander and D. A. Dixon, Resorption of glucose, fructose and meso-inositol by the foetal and post-natal sheep kidney, *J Physiol (London)* 167:480, 1963.

79. M. C. Hurd, Observations on the storage of trypan blue in the embryo chick, *Amer J Anat* 42:155, 1928.

80. C. J. Sandstrom, The storage of trypan blue in hetero-plastic chorio-allantoic grafts of embryonic duck kidney tissue, *Anat Rec* 62:7, 1935.

81. G. B. Wislocki, Experimental studies on fetal absorption. I. The vitally stained fetus, *Contrib Embryol* (no. 51) 11:45, 1920.

82. G. B. Wislocki, The fate of true solutions (phenolsulphonephthalein) and colloids (trypan blue) injected into the mammalian embryo, *Bull Johns Hopkins Hosp* 32:93, 1921.

83. W. von Möllendorff, Vitale Färbungen an tierischen Zellen, *Ergebn Physiol* 18:141, 1920.

84. J. S. Baxter and J. M. Yoffey, The post-natal development of renal tubules in the rat, *J Anat* 82:189, 1948.

85. G. C. Priestley and R. A. Malt, Development of the metanephric kidney. Protein and nucleic acid synthesis, *J Cell Biol* 37:703, 1968.

86. M. B. Burg and J. Orloff, Oxygen consumption and active transport in separated renal tubules, *Amer J Physiol* 203:327, 1962.

87. K. C. Huang and D. S. T. Lin, Kinetic studies on transport of PAH and other organic acids in isolated renal tubules, *Amer J Physiol* 208:391, 1965.

88. L. Murthy and E. C. Foulkes, Movement of solutes across luminal cell membranes in kidney tubules of the rabbit, *Nature (London)* 213:180, 1967.

89. A. Kleinzeller, K. Kolínská, and L. Beneš, Transport of glucose and galactose in kidney-cortex cells. *Biochem J* 104:843, 1967.

90. R. E. Hillman, I. Albrecht, and L. E. Rosenberg, Transport of amino acids by isolated renal tubules, *Biochim Biophys Acta* 150:528, 1968.

CHAPTER 2. DEVELOPMENT OF RENAL FUNCTION IN UTERO

1. J. Needham, *Chemical Embryology* (Cambridge: Cambridge University Press, 1931), vol. 1, p. 107.

2. Sabrazès and Fauquet, Propriétés hématolytiques de la première urine du nouveau-né, *C R Soc Biol (Paris)* 53:372, 1901.

3. A. W. Makepeace, F. Fremont-Smith, M. E. Dailey, and M. P. Carroll, The nature of the amniotic fluid, *Surg Gynec Obstet* 53:635, 1931.

4. D. P. Alexander and D. A. Nixon, The foetal kidney, *Brit Med Bull* 17:112, 1961.

5. R. L. Vernier and F. G. Smith, Jr., Fetal and neonatal kidney, in *Biology of Gestation,* ed. N. S. Assali (New York: Academic Press, 1968), vol. 2, chap. 5.

6. I. Gersh, The correlation of structure and function in the developing mesonephros and metanephros, *Contrib Embryol* (no. 153) 26:35, 1937.

7. D. L. Hutchinson, M. J. Gray, A. A. Plentl, H. Alvarez, R. Caldeyro-Barcia, B. Kaplan, and J. Lind, The role of the fetus in the water exchange of the amniotic fluid of normal and hydramniotic patients, *J Clin Invest* 38:971, 1959.

8. G. Cameron and R. Chambers, Direct evidence of function in kidney of an early human fetus, *Amer J Physiol* 123:482, 1938.

9. B. M. Patten, *Human Embryology,* ed. 3 (New York: McGraw-Hill Book Company, 1968), p. 451.

10. J. L. Bremer, The interrelations of the mesonephros, kidney and placenta in different classes of animals, *Amer J Anat* 19:179, 1916.

11. M. W. Stanier, The function of the mammalian mesonephros, *J Physiol (London)* 151:472, 1960.

12. J. S. Perry and M. W. Stanier, The rate of flow of urine of foetal pigs, *J Physiol (London)* 161:344, 1962.

13. J. Davies, Correlated anatomical and histochemical studies on the mesonephros and placenta of the sheep, *Amer J Anat* 91:263, 1952.

14. D. P. Alexander, D. A. Nixon, W. F. Widdas, and F. X. Wohlzogen, Gestational variations in the composition of the foetal fluids and foetal urine in the sheep, *J Physiol (London)* 140:1, 1958.

15. D. P. Alexander, D. A. Nixon, W. F. Widdas, and F. X. Wohlzogen, Renal function in the sheep foetus, *J Physiol (London)* 140:14, 1958.

16. R. A. McCance and M. W. Stanier, The function of the metanephros of foetal rabbits and pigs, *J Physiol (London)* 151:479, 1960.

17. R. A. McCance and E. M. Widdowson, Renal function before birth, *Proc Roy Soc London (Biol)* 141:488, 1953.

18. R. L. Vernier and A. Birch-Andersen, Studies of the human fetal kidney. I. Development of the glomerulus, *J Pediat* 60:754, 1962.

19. A. Rapoport, T. F. Nicholson, and E. R. Yendt, Movement of electrolytes across the wall of the urinary bladder in dogs, *Amer J Physiol* 198:191, 1960.

20. J. W. Boylan, E. P. Colbourn, and R. A. McCance, Renal function in the foetal and new-born guinea-pig, *J Physiol (London)* 141:323, 1958.

21. D. P. Alexander and D. A. Nixon, Plasma clearance of p-aminohippuric acid by the kidneys of foetal, neonatal and adult sheep, *Nature (London)* 194:483, 1962.

22. D. P. Alexander and D. A. Nixon, Creatinine secretion by the foetal sheep kidney (abst.), *J Physiol (London)* 171:54P, 1964.

23. J. Davies and D. V. Davies, The development of the mesonephros of the sheep, *Proc Zool Soc London* 120:73, 1950.

24. F. G. Smith, Jr., F. H. Adams, M. Borden, and J. Hilburn, Studies of renal function in the intact fetal lamb, *Amer J Obstet Gynec* 96:240, 1966.

25. M. New, H. McNamara, and N. Kretchmer, Accumulation of para-aminohippurate by slices of kidney from rabbits of various ages, *Proc Soc Exp Biol Med* 102:558, 1959.

26. B. Rennick, B. Hamilton, and R. Evans, Development of renal tubular transports of TEA and PAH in the puppy and piglet, *Amer J Physiol* 201:743, 1961.

27. N. S. Assali, G. A. Bekey, and L. W. Morrison, Fetal and neonatal circulation, in *Biology of Gestation,* ed. N. S. Assali (New York: Academic Press, 1968), vol. 2, chap. 2.

28. A. M. Rudolph and M. A. Heymann, The circulation of the fetus in utero: methods for studying distribution of blood flow, cardiac output and organ blood flow, *Circ Res* 21:163, 1967.

29. G. Meschia, J. R. Cotter, E. L. Makowski, and D. H. Barron, Simultaneous measurement of uterine and umbilical blood flows and oxygen uptakes, *Quart J Exp Physiol* 52:1, 1967.

30. A. J. Margolis and R. E. Orcutt, Pressures in human umbilical vessels in utero, *Amer J Obstet Gynec* 80:573, 1960.

31. H. Heller and E. J. Zaimis, The antidiuretic and oxytocic hormones in the posterior pituitary glands of newborn infants and adults, *J Physiol (London)* 109:162, 1949.

32. E. Diczfalusy and P. Troen, Endocrine functions of the human placenta, *Vitamins and Hormones (NY)* 19:229, 1961.

33. D. P. Alexander and D. A. Nixon, Reabsorption of glucose, fructose and meso-inositol by foetal and post-natal sheep kidney, *J Physiol (London)* 167:480, 1963.

34. I. H. Kaiser, The significance of fetal acidosis, *Amer J Obstet Gynec* 77:573, 1959.

35. T. Spackman, F. Fuchs, and N. S. Assali, Acid-base status of the fetus in human pregnancy, *Obstet Gynec* 22:785, 1963.

36. J. N. Blechner, G. Meschia, and D. H. Barron, A study of the acid-base balance of fetal sheep and goats, *Quart J Exp Physiol* 45:60, 1960.

37. D. Vaughn, T. H. Kirschbaum, T. Bersentes, P. V. Dilts, Jr., and N. S. Assali, Fetal and neonatal response to acid loading in the sheep, *J Appl Physiol* 24:135, 1968.

38. N. S. Assali, J. A. Morris, and R. Beck, Cardiovascular hemodynamics in the fetal lamb before and after lung expansion, *Amer J Physiol* 208:122, 1965.

39. F. G. Smith and A. Schwartz, Response of the intact lamb fetus to acidosis, *Amer J Obstet Gynec* 106:52, 1970.

40. F. G. Smith, Jr., B. Tinglof, and F. H. Adams, Renal phosphate clearance and bicarbonate excretion in the fetal lamb (abst.), *J Pediat* 67:944, 1965.

41. R. Day and J. Franklin, Renal carbonic anhydrase in premature and mature infants, *Pediatrics* 7:182, 1951.

42. R. A. McCance and E. M. Widdowson, Mineral metabolism of the foetus and new-born, *Brit Med Bull* 17:132, 1961.

43. W. W. McCrory, C. W. Forman, H. McNamara, and H. L. Barnett, Renal excretion of inorganic phosphate in newborn infants, *J Clin Invest* 31:357, 1952.

44. F. Fuchs and A.-R. Fuchs, Studies on the placental transfer of phosphate in the guinea pig. II. The transfer from foetus to mother, *Acta Physiol Scand* 38:391, 1957.

45. H. S. McGaughey, Jr., E. L. Corey, W. A. Scoggin, O. B. Bobbitt, Jr., and

W. N. Thornton, Jr., Observations on the equilibration of urea between mother and fetus, *Amer J Obstet Gynec* 78:844, 1959.

46. T. N. A. Jeffcoate and J. S. Scott, Polyhydramnios and oligohydramnios, *Canad Med Assn J* 80:77, 1959.

47. N. S. Assali, P. V. Dilts, Jr., A. A. Plentl, T. H. Kirschbaum, and S. J. Gross, Physiology of the placenta, in *Biology of Gestation,* ed. N. S. Assali (New York: Academic Press, 1968), vol. 1, p. 275.

48. P. D. Bruns, R. O. Linder, V. E. Drose, and F. Battaglia, The placental transfer of water from fetus to mother following the intravenous infusion of hypertonic mannitol to the maternal rabbit, *Amer J Obstet Gynec* 86:160, 1963.

49. G. D. Phillips and S. K. Sundaram, Sodium depletion of pregnant ewes and its effects on foetuses and foetal fluids, *J Physiol (London)* 184:889, 1966.

50. A. E. Seeds, Jr., Water metabolism of the fetus, *Amer J Obstet Gynec* 92:727, 1965.

51. L. M. Hellman, L. B. Flexner, W. S. Wilde, G. J. Vosburgh, and N. K. Proctor, The permeability of the human placenta to water and the supply of water to the human fetus as determined with deuterium oxide, *Amer J Obstet Gynec* 56:861, 1948.

52. D. L. Hutchinson, W. T. Kelly, E. A. Friedman, and A. A. Plentl, The distribution and metabolism of carbon-labeled urea in pregnant primates, *J Clin Invest* 41:1745, 1962.

53. G. Wagner and F. Fuchs, The volume of amniotic fluid in the first half of human pregnancy, *J Obstet Gynaec Brit Comm* 69:131, 1962.

54. P. N. Gillibrand, Changes in amniotic fluid volume with advancing pregnancy, *J Obstet Gynaec Brit Comm* 76:527, 1969.

55. P. N. Gillibrand, The rate of water transfer from the amniotic sac with advancing pregnancy, *J Obstet Gynaec Brit Comm* 76:530, 1969.

56. R. L. Gadd, The volume of the liquor amnii in normal and abnormal pregnancies, *J Obstet Gynaec Brit Comm* 73:11, 1966.

57. R. M. Pitkin and S. J. Zwirek, Amniotic fluid creatinine, *Amer J Obstet Gynec* 98:1135, 1967.

58. P. A. Miles and J. W. Pearson, Amniotic fluid osmolality in assessing fetal maturity, *Obstet Gynec* 34:701, 1969.

59. A. C. Barnes, *Intra-Uterine Development* (Philadelphia: Lea & Febiger, 1968), p. 136.

60. A. D. Bain and J. S. Scott, Renal agenesis and severe urinary tract dysplasia: a review of 50 cases, with particular reference to the associated anomalies, *Brit Med J* 1:841, 1960.

61. W. W. McCrory, unpublished observations.

62. J. M. Evanson and S. W. Stanbury, Congenital chloridorrhoea or so-called congenital alkalosis and diarrhoea, *Gut* 6:29, 1965.

63. J. A. Pritchard, Deglutition by normal and anencephalic fetuses, *Obstet Gynec* 25:289, 1965.

64. R. A. Chez, F. G. Smith, and D. L. Hutchinson, Renal function in the intrauterine primate fetus. I. Experimental technique; rate of formation and chemical composition of urine, *Amer J Obstet Gynec* 90:128, 1964.

CHAPTER 3. QUANTITATIVE MEASUREMENT OF RENAL FUNCTION DURING GROWTH IN INFANCY AND CHILDHOOD

1. J. T. Oliver, M. Rubenstein, R. Meyer, and J. Bernstein, Congenital abnormalities of the urinary system. III. Growth of the kidney in childhood—determination of normal weight, *J Pediat* 61:256, 1962.

2. J. M. Coppoletta and S. B. Wolbach, Body length and organ weights of infants and children: a study of the body length and normal weights of the more important organs of the body between birth and twelve years of age, *Amer J Path* 9:55, 1933.

3. C. J. Hodson, J. A. Drewe, M. N. Karn, and A. King, Renal size in normal children. A radiographic study during life, *Arch Dis Child* 37:616, 1962.

4. O. M. B. Gatewood, R. J. Glasser, and J. J. Vanhoutte, Roentgen evaluation of renal size in pediatric age groups, *Amer J Dis Child* 110:162, 1965.

5. F. Walter and T. Addis, Organ work and organ weight, *J Exp Med* 69:467, 1939.

6. D. Potter, A. Jarrah, T. Sakai, J. Harrah, and M. A. Holliday, Character of function and size in kidney during normal growth of rats, *Pediat Res* 3:51, 1969.

7. H. W. Smith, *Principles of Renal Physiology* (New York: Oxford University Press, 1956).

8. H. L. Barnett, Kidney function in young infants, *Pediatrics* 5:171, 1950.

9. R. F. Pitts, *Physiology of the Kidney and Body Fluids,* ed. 2 (Chicago: Year Book Medical Publishers, Inc., 1968), p. 64.

10. M. L. Cohen, F. G. Smith, Jr., R. S. Mindell, and R. L. Vernier, A simple, reliable method of measuring glomerular filtration rate using single, low dose sodium iothalamate I^{131}, *Pediatrics* 43:407, 1969.

11. T. Sakai, E. P. Leumann, and M. A. Holliday, Single injection clearance in children, *Pediatrics* 44:905, 1969.

12. I. M. L. Donaldson, Comparison of the renal clearances of inulin and radioactive diatrizoate ("Hypaque") as measures of the glomerular filtration rate in man, *Clin Sci* 35:513, 1968.

13. L. A. Sapirstein, D. G. Vidt, M. J. Mandel, and G. Hanusek, Volumes of distribution and clearances of intravenously injected creatinine in the dog, *Amer J Physiol* 181:330, 1955.

14. B. Truniger, A. Donath, and M. Kappeler, Simplified clearance techniques: the single injection method and its modifications, *Helv Med Acta* 34:116, 1968.

15. Pitts, note 9, p. 144.

16. A. C. Barger and J. A. Herd, The renal circulation, *New Eng J Med* 284:482, 1971.

17. G. D. Thorburn, H. H. Kopald, and J. A. Herd, Intrarenal distribution of nutrient blood flow determined with krypton^{85} in the unanesthetized dog, *Circ Res* 13:290, 1963.

18. E. E. Windhager, J. E. Lewy, and A. Spitzer, Intrarenal control of proximal tubular reabsorption of sodium and water, *Nephron* 6:247, 1969.

19. M. H. Maxwell, E. S. Breed, and H. W. Smith, Significance of the renal juxtamedullary circulation in man, *Amer J Med* 9:216, 1950.

20. L. A. Pilkington, R. Binder, J. C. M. de Haas, and R. F. Pitts, Intrarenal distribution of blood flow, *Amer J Physiol* 208:1107, 1965.

21. M. Horster and K. Thurau, Micropuncture studies on the filtration rate of single superficial and juxtamedullary glomeruli in the rat kidney, *Pflueger Arch Ges Physiol* 301:162, 1968.

22. G. H. Fetterman, N. A. Shuplock, F. J. Philipp, and H. S. Gregg, The growth and maturation of human glomeruli and proximal convolutions from term to adulthood: studies by microdissection, *Pediatrics* 35:601, 1965.

23. P. L. Calcagno and M. I. Rubin, Renal extraction of para-aminohippurate in infants and children, *J Clin Invest* 42:1632, 1963.

24. M. Horster and J. E. Lewy, Filtration fraction and extraction of PAH during neonatal period in the rat, *Amer J Physiol* 219:1061, 1970.

25. M. Horster and H. Valtin, Postnatal development of renal function: micropuncture and clearance studies in the dog, *J Clin Invest* 50:779, 1971.

26. P. A. Jose, A. G. Logan, L. M. Slotkoff, L. S. Lilienfield, P. L. Calcagno, and G. M. Eisner, Intrarenal blood flow distribution in canine puppies, *Pediat Res* 5:335, 1971.

27. Pitts, note 9, p. 129.

28. Ibid., p. 73.

29. S. E. Bradley, J. H. Laragh, H. O. Wheeler, ·M. MacDowell, and J. Oliver, Correlation of structure and function in the handling of glucose by the nephrons of the canine kidney, *J Clin Invest* 40:1113, 1961.

30. R. E. Rieselbach, S. W. Shankel, E. Slatopolsky, H. Lubowitz, and N. S. Bricker, Glucose titration studies in patients with chronic progressive renal disease, *J Clin Invest* 46:157, 1967.

31. H. L. Barnett, W. K. Hare, H. McNamara, and R. S. Hare, Influence of postnatal age on kidney function of premature infants, *Proc Soc Exp Biol Med* 69:55, 1948.

32. M. I. Rubin, E. Bruck, and M. Rapoport, Maturation of renal function in childhood: clearance studies, *J Clin Invest* 28:1144, 1949.

33. M. Pérez-Stable, La prueba de inulina en niños normales; medida del filtrado glomerular, *Arch med inf* 16:89, 1947.

34. F. Tudvad and J. Vesterdal, The maximal tubular transfer of glucose and para-amino-hippurate in premature infants, *Acta Paediat* 42:337, 1953.

35. F. K. Friederiszick, Nieren-Clearance-Untersuchungen im Kindesalter, *Bibl Paediat* suppl. 57, 1954.

36. R. F. A. Dean and R. A. McCance, Inulin, diodone, creatinine and urea clearances in newborn infants, *J Physiol (London)* 106:431, 1947.

37. J. R. West, H. W. Smith, and H. Chasis, Glomerular filtration rate, effective renal blood flow, and maximal tubular excretory capacity in infancy, *J Pediat* 32:10, 1948.

38. E. L. Potter and S. T. Thierstein, Glomerular development in the kidney as an index of fetal maturity, *J Pediat* 22:695, 1943.

39. M. S. Macdonald and J. L. Emery, The late intrauterine and postnatal development of human renal glomeruli, *J Anat* 93:331, 1959.

40. R. L. Jamison, Micropuncture study of superficial proximal tubules, juxtamedullary loops of Henle and papillary segments of the collecting duct of the young rat kidney (abst.), *Proc 4th Int Cong Nephrol,* Stockholm, 1969, p. 242.

41. J. Lind and C. Wegelius, Human fetal circulation: changes in the cardiovascular system at birth and disturbances in the postnatal closure of the foramen ovale and ductus arteriosus, *Cold Spring Harbor Symposia Quant Biol* 19:109, 1954.

42. A. M. Rappaport, discussion cited in *Fetal and Infant Liver Function and Structure, Ann NY Acad Sci* 111:527, 1963.

43. W. Oh, M. A. Oh, and J. Lind, Renal function and blood volume in the newborn infant related to placental transfusion, *Acta Paediat Scand* 56:197, 1966.

44. E. Y. Berger, S. J. Farber, and D. P. Earle, Jr., Renal excretion of mannitol, *Proc Soc Exp Biol Med* 66:62, 1947.

45. W. W. McCrory, C. W. Forman, H. McNamara, and H. L. Barnett, Renal excretion of inorganic phosphate in newborn infants, *J Clin Invest* 31:357, 1952.

46. J. B. Richmond, H. Kravitz, W. Segar, and H. A. Waisman, Renal clearance of endogenous phosphate in infants and children, *Proc Soc Exp Biol Med* 77:83, 1951.

47. J. M. Tanner, R. M. Whitehouse, and M. Takaishi, Standards from birth to maturity for height, weight, height velocity and weight velocity: British children, 1965. Parts I and II, *Arch Dis Child* 41:454 and 613, 1966.

48. D. H. Weintraub, P. L. Calcagno, M. K. Kelleher, and M. I. Rubin, Mechanism of renal glycosuria in ACTH-treated premature infants, *Proc Soc Exp Biol Med* 81:542, 1952.

49. E. Galán, M. Pérez-Stable, J. Más Martín, and O. García Faez, Las pruebas renales de aclaramiento y saturación en el niño normal, *Arch med inf* 16:102, 1947.

50. C. M. Edelmann, Jr. and J. Bernstein, The kidneys and urinary tract, in *Pediatrics,* ed. 14, ed. H. L. Barnett and A. H. Einhorn (New York: Appleton-Century-Crofts, 1968), chap. 24, p. 1332.

51. J. Winberg, The 24-hour true endogenous creatinine clearance in infants and children without renal disease, *Acta Paediat* 48:443, 1959.

52. G. Mattar, H. L. Barnett, H. McNamara, and H. D. Lauson, Measurement of glomerular filtration rate in children with kidney disease, *J Clin Invest* 31:938, 1952.

53. R. S. Hare, Endogenous creatinine in serum and urine, *Proc Soc Exp Biol Med* 74:148, 1950.

54. B. Kuhlbäck, A. Pasternack, K. Launiala, and M. Stenberg, Serum creatine and creatinine in children and adolescents, *Scand J Clin Lab Invest* 22:37, 1968.

55. K. Hare, H. Goldstein, H. L. Barnett, H. McNamara, and R. S. Hare, Renal excretion of creatinine in man (abst.), *Fed Proc* 8:67, 1949.

56. W. F. Dodge, L. B. Travis, and C. W. Daeschner, Comparison of endogenous creatinine clearance with inulin clearance, *Amer J Dis Child* 113:683, 1967.

57. M. New, H. McNamara, and N. Kretchmer, Accumulation of para-aminohip-

purate by slices of kidney from rabbits of various ages, *Proc Soc Exp Biol Med* 102:558, 1959.

58. B. Rennick, B. Hamilton, and R. Evans, Development of renal tubular transports of TEA and PAH in the puppy and piglet, *Amer J Physiol* 201:743, 1961.

59. J. S. Baxter and J. M. Yoffey, The post-natal development of renal tubules in the rat, *J Anat* 82:189, 1948.

60. G. C. Priestley and R. A. Malt, Development of the metanephric kidney: protein and nucleic acid synthesis, *J Cell Biol* 37:703, 1968.

61. Pitts, note 9, p. 228.

62. D. F. Davies and N. W. Shock, Age changes in glomerular filtration rate, effective renal plasma flow, and tubular secretory capacity in adult males, *J Clin Invest* 29:496, 1950.

63. J. M. Tanner, Fallacy of per-weight and per-surface area standards and their relation to spurious correlation, *J Appl Physiol* 2:1, 1949.

64. P. L. Calcagno and M. I. Rubin, Effect of dehydration produced by water deprivation, diarrhea and vomiting on renal function in infants, *Pediatrics* 7:328, 1951.

65. R. A. McCance and E. M. Widdowson, The correct physiological basis on which to compare infant and adult renal function, *Lancet* ii:860, 1952.

66. B. Friis-Hansen, Changes in body water compartments during growth, *Acta Paediat* 46:suppl. 110, 1957.

67. I. S. Edelman, H. B. Haley, P. R. Schloerb, D. B. Sheldon, B. J. Friis-Hansen, G. Stoll, and F. D. Moore, Further observations on total body water. I. Normal values throughout the life span, *Surg Gynec Obstet* 95:1, 1952.

68. E. M. Darmady, J. Offer, J. Prince, and F. Stranack, The proximal convoluted tubule in the renal handling of water, *Lancet* ii:1254, 1964.

69. E. M. Darmady, personal communication.

70. J. Oliver and M. MacDowell, The structural and functional aspects of the handling of glucose by the nephrons and the kidney and their correlation by means of structural-functional equivalents, *J Clin Invest* 40:1093, 1961.

71. H. W. Smith, *Lectures on the Kidney* (Lawrence, Kansas: University of Kansas, 1943), p. 104.

72. V. Osathanondh and E. L. Potter, Development of the human kidney as shown by microdissection. I. Preparation of tissue with reasons for possible misinterpretation of observations, *Arch Path (Chicago)* 76:271, 1963.

73. H. Elias and A. Hennig, Stereology of the human renal glomerulus, in *Quantitative Methods in Morphology,* ed. E. R. Weibel and H. Elias (New York: Springer-Verlag, 1967), p. 131.

74. G. H. Fetterman, personal communication.

75. M. Horster, B. J. Kemler, and H. Valtin, Intracortical distribution of number and volume of glomeruli during postnatal maturation in the dog, *J Clin Invest* 50:796, 1971.

76. N. S. Bricker, S. Klahr, H. Lubowitz, and R. E. Rieselbach, Renal function in chronic renal disease, *Medicine (Balt)* 44:263, 1965.

77. W. S. Kerr, Jr., Effect of complete ureteral obstruction in dogs on kidney function, *Amer J Physiol* 184:521, 1956.

78. W. Suki, G. Eknoyan, F. C. Rector, Jr., and D. W. Seldin, Patterns of nephron perfusion in acute and chronic hydronephrosis, *J Clin Invest* 45:122, 1966.

79. J. P. Hayslett, M. Kashgarian, and F. H. Epstein, Functional correlates of compensatory renal hypertrophy, *J Clin Invest* 47:774, 1968.

80. A. I. Katz and F. H Epstein, Relation of glomerular filtration rate and sodium reabsorption to kidney size in compensatory renal hypertrophy, *Yale J Biol Med* 40:222, 1967.

81. K. Čapek, H. Dlouhá, and M. Kubát, The development of proximal tubular function in young rats (micropuncture study) (abst.), *Proc 4th Int Cong Nephrol,* Stockholm, 1969, p. 244.

82. E. E. Arrizurieta De Muchnik, E. M. Lipham, and C. W. Gottschalk, Form and function in normal and hypertrophied nephrons, in *Compensatory Renal Hypertrophy,* ed. W. W. Nowinski and R. J. Goss (New York: Academic Press, 1969), p. 29.

83. R. J. Goss, *Adaptive Growth* (London: Logos Press Ltd., 1964).

CHAPTER 4. RENAL FUNCTION IN THE POSTNATAL PERIOD

1. S. A. Doxiadis, M. K. Goldfinch, and N. Cole, "Proteinuria" in the newborn, *Lancet* ii:1242, 1952.

2. P. G. Rhodes, C. L. Hammel, and L. B. Berman, Urinary constituents of the newborn infant, *J Pediat* 60:18, 1962.

3. M. F. Randolph and M. Greenfield, Proteinuria. A six-year study of normal infants, preschool and school age populations previously screened for urinary tract disease, *Amer J Dis Child* 114:631, 1967.

4. K. Lincoln and J. Winberg, Studies of urinary tract infections in infancy and childhood. III. Quantitative estimation of cellular excretion in unselected neonates, *Acta Paediat* 53:447, 1964.

5. H. Silver, J. C. Drever, and D. M. Douglas, Cells in the urine of newborn infants, *Arch Dis Child* 42:598, 1967.

6. G. Cruickshank and E. Edmond, "Clean catch" urines in the newborn. Bacteriology and cell excretion patterns in first week of life, *Brit Med J* 4:705, 1967.

7. C. V. Pryles, Percutaneous bladder aspiration and other methods of urine collection for bacteriologic study, *Pediatrics* 36:128, 1965.

8. W. T. Weathers and J. E. Wenzl, Suprapubic aspiration of the bladder. Perforation of a viscus other than the bladder, *Amer J Dis Child* 117:590, 1969.

9. J. M. Stansfeld and J. K. G. Webb, Observations on pyuria in children, *Arch Dis Child* 28:386, 1953.

10. R. F. Pitts, *Physiology of the Kidney and Body Fluids,* ed. 2 (Chicago: Year Book Medical Publishers, Inc., 1968), p. 94.

11. H. Wirz, B. Hargitay, and W. Kuhn, Lokalisation des Konzentrierungsprozesses in der Niere durch direkte Kryoskopie, *Helv Physiol Pharmacol Acta* 9:196, 1951.

12. R. W. Berliner and D. G. Davidson, Production of hypertonic urine in the absence of pituitary antidiuretic hormone, *J Clin Invest* 36:1416, 1957.

13. Pitts, note 10, p. 101.

14. E. L. Pratt and S. E. Snyderman, Renal water requirement of infants fed evaporated milk with and without added carbohydrates, *Pediatrics* 11:65, 1953.

15. J. Winberg, Determination of renal concentration capacity in infants and children without renal disease, *Acta Paediat* 48:318, 1959.

16. E. Poláček, J. Vocel, L. Neugebauerová, M. Šebková, and E. Věchetová, The osmotic concentrating ability in healthy infants and children, *Arch Dis Child* 40:291, 1965.

17. P. L. Calcagno, M. I. Rubin, and D. H. Weintraub, Studies on the renal concentrating and diluting mechanisms in the premature infant, *J Clin Invest* 33:91, 1954.

18. C. M. Edelmann, Jr., H. L. Barnett, and V. Troupkou, Renal concentrating mechanisms in newborn infants. Effects of dietary protein and water content, role of urea, and responsiveness to antidiuretic hormone, *J Clin Invest* 39:1062, 1960.

19. G. H. Fleischaker, O. J. Gesink, and W. W. McCrory, Effect of age on distribution of urea and electrolyte in kidneys of young rabbits (abst.), *Amer J Dis Child* 100:557, 1960.

20. J. N. Forrest, Jr. and M. W. Stanier, Kidney composition and renal concentration ability in young rabbits, *J Physiol (London)* 187:1, 1966.

21. P. Yunibhand and U. Held, Nierenmark und Urinosmolalität nach der Geburt bei der Ratte unter Flüssigkeitsentzug, *Helv Physiol Pharmacol Acta* 23:91, 1965.

22. J. M. N. Boss, H. Dlouhá, M. Kraus, and J. Křeček, The structure of the kidney in relation to age and diet in white rats during the weaning period, *J Physiol (London)* 168:196, 1963.

23. H. Heller, The renal function of newborn infants, *J Physiol (London)* 102:429, 1944.

24. H. Heller, The water metabolism of newborn infants and animals, *Arch Dis Child* 26:195, 1951.

25. H. Heller and E. J. Zaimis, The antidiuretic and oxytocic hormones in the posterior pituitary glands of newborn infants and adults, *J Physiol (London)* 109:162, 1949.

26. M. Janovský, J. Martínek, and V. Stanincová, Antidiuretic activity in the plasma of human infants after a load of sodium chloride, *Acta Paediat Scand* 54:543, 1965.

27. J. P. Connelly, J. D. Crawford, and J. Watson, Studies of neonatal hyperphosphatemia, *Pediatrics* 30:425, 1962.

28. R. A. McCance and E. M. Widdowson, Renal function before birth, *Proc Roy Soc (Biol)* 141:488, 1953.

29. C. A. Smith, S. Yudkin, W. Young, A. Minkowski, and M. Cushman, Adjustment of electrolytes and water following premature birth (with special reference to edema), *Pediatrics* 3:34, 1949.

30. R. G. Ames, Urinary water excretion and neurohypophysial function in full term and premature infants shortly after birth, *Pediatrics* 12:272, 1953.

31. H. L. Barnett, J. Vesterdal, H. McNamara, and H. D. Lauson, Renal water excretion in premature infants, *J Clin Invest* 31:1069, 1952.

32. F. H. Epstein, C. R. Kleeman, S. Pursel, and A. Hendrikx, The effect of feeding protein and urea on the renal concentrating process, *J Clin Invest* 36:635, 1957.

33. C. M. Edelmann, Jr., H. L. Barnett, and H. Stark, Effect of urea on concentration of urinary nonurea solute in premature infants, *J Appl Physiol* 21:1021, 1966.

34. R. A. McCance and E. M. Widdowson, Mineral metabolism of the foetus and new-born, *Brit Med Bull* 17:132, 1961.

35. C. M. Edelmann, Jr., H. L. Barnett, H. Stark, H. Boichis, and J. R. Soriano, A standardized test of renal concentrating capacity in children, *Amer J Dis Child* 114:639, 1967.

36. D. C. Darrow, R. E. Cooke, and W. E. Segar, Water and electrolyte metabolism in infants fed cow's milk mixtures during heat stress, *Pediatrics* 14:602, 1954.

37. P. A. Hoy, Diuresis in newborn rat given intravenous water or salt solution, *Proc Soc Exp Biol Med* 122:358, 1966.

38. H. I. Goldman, S. Karelitz, H. Acs, and E. Seifter, The relationship of the sodium, potassium, and chloride concentration of the feeding to the weight gain of premature infants, *Pediatrics* 30:909, 1962.

39. L. Finberg and H. E. Harrison, Hypernatremia in infants. An evaluation of the clinical and biochemical findings accompanying this state, *Pediatrics* 16:1, 1955.

40. R. F. A. Dean and R. A. McCance, The renal responses of infants and adults to the administration of hypertonic solutions of sodium chloride and urea, *J Physiol (London)* 109:81, 1949.

41. G. Giebisch, Functional organization of proximal and distal tubular electrolyte transport, *Nephron* 6:260, 1969.

42. L. E. Early, J. A. Martino, and R. M. Friedler, Factors affecting sodium reabsorption by the proximal tubule as determined during blockade of distal sodium reabsorption, *J Clin Invest* 45:1668, 1966.

43. E. E. Windhager, Glomerulo-tubular balance of salt and water, *Physiologist* 11:103, 1968.

44. K. M. Koch, H. S. Aynedjian, and N. Bank, Effect of acute hypertension on sodium reabsorption by the proximal tubule, *J Clin Invest* 47:1696, 1968.

45. C. M. Edelmann, Jr., Maturation of the neonatal kidney, in *Proc 3rd Int Cong Nephrol, Washington, 1966* (New York: S. Karger, 1967), vol. 3, p. 1.

46. J. H. Dirks, W. J. Cirksena, and R. W. Berliner, The effect of saline infusion on sodium reabsorption by the proximal tubule of the dog, *J Clin Invest* 44:1160, 1965.

47. M. A. Cortney, M. Mylle, W. E. Lassiter, and C. W. Gottschalk, Renal tubular transport of water, solute, and PAH in rats loaded with isotonic saline, *Amer J Physiol* 209:1199, 1965.

48. A. J. Greenberg, H. McNamara, and W. W. McCrory, Renal tubular response to aldosterone in normal infants and children with adrenal disorders, *J Clin Endocr* 27:1197, 1967.

49. Pitts, note 10, p. 180.

50. R. F. Pitts, J. L. Ayer, and W. A. Schiess, The renal regulation of acid-base

balance in man. III. The reabsorption and excretion of bicarbonate, *J Clin Invest* 28:35, 1949.

51. F. C. Rector, Jr., N. W. Carter, and D. W. Seldin, The mechanism of bicarbonate reabsorption in the proximal and distal tubules of the kidney, *J Clin Invest* 44:278, 1965.

52. F. C. Rector, Jr., D. W. Seldin, A. D. Roberts, Jr., and J. S. Smith, The role of plasma CO_2 tension and carbonic anhydrase activity in the renal reabsorption of bicarbonate, *J Clin Invest* 39:1706, 1960.

53. M. L. Purkerson, H. Lubowitz, R. W. White, and N. S. Bricker, On the influence of extracellular fluid volume expansion on bicarbonate reabsorption in the rat, *J Clin Invest* 48:1754, 1969.

54. J. R. Soriano, H. Boichis, H. Stark, and C. M. Edelmann, Jr., Proximal renal tubular acidosis. A defect in bicarbonate reabsorption with normal urinary acidification, *Pediat Res* 1:81, 1967.

55. R. C. Morris, Jr., An experimental renal acidification defect in patients with hereditary fructose intolerance. II. Its distinction from classical renal tubular acidosis; its resemblance to the renal acidification defect associated with the Fanconi syndrome of children with cystinosis, *J Clin Invest* 47:1648, 1968.

56. F. H. Tudvad, H. McNamara, and H. L. Barnett, Renal response of premature infants to administration of bicarbonate and potassium, *Pediatrics* 13:4, 1954.

57. C. M. Edelmann, Jr., J. R. Soriano, H. Boichis, A. B. Gruskin, and M. I. Acosta, Renal bicarbonate reabsorption and hydrogen ion excretion in normal infants, *J Clin Invest* 46:1309, 1967.

58. M. S. Albert and R. W. Winters, Acid-base equilibrium of blood in normal infants, *Pediatrics* 37:728, 1966.

59. A. Peonides, B. Levin, and W. F. Young, The renal excretion of hydrogen ions in infants and children, *Arch Dis Child* 40:33, 1965.

60. C. M. Edelmann, Jr., H. Boichis, J. R. Soriano, and H. Stark, The renal response of children to acute ammonium chloride acidosis, *Pediat Res* 1:452, 1967.

61. W. A. Schiess, J. L. Ayer, W. D. Lotspeich, and R. F. Pitts, The renal regulation of acid-base balance in man. II. Factors affecting the excretion of titratable acid by the normal human subject, *J Clin Invest* 27:57, 1948.

62. A. S. Relman, Renal acidosis and renal excretion of acid in health and disease, in *Advances in Internal Medicine*, ed. W. Dock and I. Snapper (Chicago: Year Book Medical Publishers, Inc., 1964), vol. 12, p. 295.

63. S. J. Fomon, D. M. Harris, and R. L. Jensen, Acidification of the urine by infants fed human milk and whole cow's milk, *Pediatrics* 23:113, 1959.

64. N. Hatemi and R. A. McCance, Renal aspects of acid-base control in the newly born. III. Response to acidifying drugs, *Acta Paediat* 50:603, 1961.

65. Pitts, note 10, p. 75.

66. L. I. Gardner, E. A. MacLachlan, W. Pick, M. L. Terry, and A. M. Butler, Etiologic factors in tetany of newly born infants, *Pediatrics* 5:228, 1950.

67. H. Bakwin, Tetany in newborn infants: relation to physiologic hypoparathyroidism, *J Pediat* 14:1, 1939.

68. W. W. McCrory, C. W. Forman, H. McNamara, and H. L. Barnett, Renal excretion of inorganic phosphate in newborn infants, *J Clin Invest* 31:357, 1952.

69. C. Anast, Tetany of the newborn, in *Endocrine and Genetic Diseases of Childhood,* ed. L. I. Gardner (Philadelphia: W. B. Saunders Co., 1969), chap. 4, p. 352.

70. Pitts, note 10, p. 77.

71. J. B. Richmond, H. Kravitz, W. Segar, and H. A. Waisman, Renal clearance of endogenous phosphate in infants and children, *Proc Soc Exp Biol Med* 77:83, 1951.

72. R. F. A. Dean and R. A. McCance, Phosphate clearances in infants and adults, *J Physiol (London)* 107:182, 1948.

73. P. P. Lambert, E. van Kessel, and C. Leplat, Etude sur l'élimination des phosphates inorganiques chez l'homme, *Acta Med Scand* 128:386, 1947.

74. R. W. Ollayos and A. W. Winkler, Urinary excretion and serum concentration of inorganic phosphate in man, *J Clin Invest* 22:147, 1943.

75. B. E. C. Nordin and R. Fraser, Assessment of urinary phosphate excretion, *Lancet* i:947, 1960.

76. H. Janse, H. H. Van Gelderen, and J. H. Ruys, Assessment of urinary phosphate excretion in normal and abnormal children, *Arch Dis Child* 41:541, 1966.

77. P. L. Calcagno and C. U. Lowe, Substrate-induced renal tubular maturation (abst.), *J Pediat* 63:851, 1963.

78. C. M. Edelmann, Jr. and N. M. Wolfish, Dietary influence on renal maturation in premature infants (abst.), *Pediat Res* 2:421, 1968.

CHAPTER 5. CELLULAR PROCESSES UNDERLYING GROWTH AND DEVELOPMENT OF THE KIDNEY

1. R. J. Goss, *Adaptive Growth* (London: Logos Press Ltd., 1964), p. 13.

2. C. H. Smith and J. M. Kissane, Distribution of forms of lactic dehydrogenase within the developing rat kidney, *Develop Biol* 8:151, 1963.

3. M. R. Vetter and C. W. Gibley, Jr., Morphogenesis and histochemistry of the developing mouse kidney, *J Morph* 120:135, 1966.

4. A. B. O. Desalu, Correlation of localization of alkaline and acid phosphatases with morphological development of the rat kidney, *Anat Rec* 154:253, 1966.

5. V. K. Hopsu, S. Ruponen, and S. Talanti, Leucine aminopeptidase in the foetal kidney of the rat, *Experientia* 17:271, 1961.

6. G. R. Wacker, H. S. Zarkowsky, and H. B. Burch, Changes in kidney enzymes of rats after birth, *Amer J Physiol* 200:367, 1961.

7. A. Zorzoli, I. J. Turkenkopf, and V. L. Mueller, Gluconeogenesis in developing rat kidney cortex, *Biochem J* 111:181, 1969.

8. H. Krebs, Gluconeogenesis, *Proc Roy Soc (Biol)* 159:545, 1964.

9. G. H. Hirsch and J. B. Hook, Maturation of renal organic acid transport: substrate stimulation by penicillin, *Science* 165:909, 1969.

10. M. Winick and A. Noble, Quantitative changes in DNA, RNA and protein during prenatal and postnatal growth in the rat, *Develop Biol* 12:451, 1965.

11. G. C. Priestley and R. A. Malt, Development of the metanephric kidney: protein and nucleic acid synthesis, *J Cell Biol* 37:703, 1968.

12. H. D. Rollason, Growth and differentiation of the fetal kidney following bilateral nephrectomy of the pregnant rat at 18½ days of gestation, *Anat Rec* 141:183, 1961.

13. R. J. Goss, Effects of maternal nephrectomy on foetal kidneys, *Nature (London)* 198:1108, 1963.

14. R. A. Malt and D. A. Lemaitre, Nucleic acids in fetal kidney after maternal nephrectomy, *Proc Soc Exp Biol Med* 130:539, 1969.

15. F. Friedberg, M. P. Schulman, and D. M. Greenberg, The effect of growth on the incorporation of glycine labeled with radioactive carbon into the protein of liver homogenates, *J Biol Chem* 173:437, 1948.

16. R. J. Schain, M. J. Carver, J. H. Copenhaver, and N. R. Underdahl, Protein metabolism in the developing brain: influence of birth and gestational age, *Science* 156:984, 1967.

17. S. L. Clark, Jr., Cellular differentiation in the kidneys of newborn mice studied with the electron microscope, *J Biophys Biochem Cytol* 3:349, 1957.

18. W. W. Nowinski and R. J. Goss, eds., *Compensatory Renal Hypertrophy* (New York: Academic Press, 1969).

19. I. W. Halliburton and R. Y. Thomson, Chemical aspects of compensatory renal hypertrophy, *Cancer Res* 25:1882, 1965.

20. F. L. Coe and P. R. Korty, Protein synthesis during compensatory renal hypertrophy, *Amer J Physiol* 213:1585, 1967.

21. J. P. Hayslett, M. Kashgarian, and F. H. Epstein, Functional correlates of compensatory renal hypertrophy, *J Clin Invest* 47:774, 1968.

22. R. A. Malt and D. A. Lemaitre, Accretion and turnover of RNA in the renoprival kidney, *Amer J Physiol* 214:1041, 1968.

23. S. Marshall, Renal compensatory hypertrophy in unilateral disease of the kidney, *Int Abst Surg* 117:307, 1963.

24. G. E. G. Williams, Some aspects of compensatory hyperplasia of the kidney, *Brit J Exp Path* 42:386, 1961.

25. G. Threlfall, D. M. Taylor, and A. T. Buck, Studies of the changes in growth and DNA synthesis in the rat kidney during experimentally induced renal hypertrophy, *Amer J Path* 50:1, 1967.

26. W. A. Anderson, The fine structure of compensatory growth in the rat kidney after unilateral nephrectomy, *Amer J Anat* 121:217, 1967.

27. S. N. Rous and K. G. Wakim, Kidney function before, during and after compensatory hypertrophy, *J Urol* 98:30, 1967.

28. B. Bugge-Asperheim and F. Kiil, Examination of growth-mediated changes in hemodynamics and tubular transport of sodium, glucose and hippurate after nephrectomy, *Scand J Clin Lab Invest* 22:255, 1968.

29. A. I. Katz and F. H. Epstein, Relation of glomerular filtration rate and sodium reabsorption to kidney size in compensatory renal hypertrophy, *Yale J Biol Med* 40:222, 1967.

30. M. A. Holliday, personal communication.

31. G. Peters, Compensatory adaptation of renal functions in the unanesthetized rat, *Amer J Physiol* 205:1042, 1963.

32. J. B. Van Liew, H. Stolte, and J. W. Boylan, Micropuncture studies of proxi-

mal tubular protein reabsorption in normal and hypertrophied rat kidney (abst.), *Fed Proc* 26:375, 1967.

33. F. Walter and T. Addis, Organ work and organ weight, *J Exp Med* 69:467, 1939.

34. T. N. Pullman, A. S. Alving, R. J. Dern, and M. Landowne, The influence of dietary protein intake on specific renal functions in normal man, *J Lab Clin Med* 44:320, 1954.

35. W. D. Lotspeich, Renal hypertrophy in metabolic acidosis and its relation to ammonia excretion, *Amer J Physiol* 208:1135, 1965.

36. R. J. Goss and M. Rankin, Physiological factors affecting compensatory renal hyperplasia in the rat, *J Exp Zool* 145:209, 1960.

37. J. H. Baxter and G. C. Cotzias, Effects of proteinuria on the kidney. Proteinuria, renal enlargement, and renal injury consequent on protracted parenteral administration of protein solution in rats, *J Exp Med* 89:643, 1949.

38. P. C. Royce, Role of renal uptake of plasma protein in compensatory renal hypertrophy, *Amer J Physiol* 212:924, 1967.

39. P. L. Calcagno and C. U. Lowe, Substrate-induced renal tubular maturation (abst.), *J Pediat* 63:851, 1963.

40. C. M. Edelmann, Jr. and N. M. Wolfish, Dietary influence on renal maturation in premature infants (abst.), *Pediat Res* 2:421, 1968.

41. R. F. Pitts, The effect of infusing glycin and of varying the dietary protein intake on renal hemodynamics in the dog, *Amer J Physiol* 142:355, 1944.

42. S. E. Dicker, Effect of the protein content of the diet on the glomerular filtration rate of young and adult rats, *J Physiol (London)* 108:197, 1949.

43. A. I. Katz and F. H. Epstein, The role of sodium-potassium-activated adenosine triphosphatase in the reabsorption of sodium by the kidney, *J Clin Invest* 46:1999, 1967.

44. W. W. Nowinski, U. Carpentieri, and W. C. Mahaffey, Glutamic dehydrogenase and alkaline phosphatase in compensatory hypertrophy of the rat kidney, *Proc Soc Exp Biol Med* 129:26, 1968.

45. J. K. Farquhar, W. N. Scott, and F. L. Coe, Hexose monophosphate shunt activity in compensatory renal hypertrophy, *Proc Soc Exp Biol Med* 129:809, 1968.

46. H. A. Johnson and F. Amendola, Mitochondrial proliferation in compensatory growth of the kidney, *Amer J Path* 54:35, 1969.

47. F. Dies and W. D. Lotspeich, Hexose monophosphate shunt in the kidney during acid-base and electrolyte imbalance, *Amer J Physiol* 212:61, 1967.

48. S. Rosenthal, I. Teichmann, and E. Winkelmann, Das Verhalten von Atmungsenzymen in hypertrophierendem Nierengewebe, *Acta Biol Med German* 8:530, 1962.

49. E. Mascitelli-Coriandoli and A. Ieranò, Ipertrofia compensatoria del rene superstite in animali nefrectomizzati. IX. Comportamento della piridossina e del piridossale-5-fosfato, *Boll Soc Ital Biol Sper* 44:1278, 1968.

50. W. W. Nowinski and A. Pigón, The Krebs cycle in glomeruli of normal rat kidney and in compensatory hypertrophy, *J Histochem Cytochem* 15:32, 1967.

51. H. A. Johnson and J. M. Vera Roman, Compensatory renal enlargement. Hypertrophy versus hyperplasia, *Amer J Path* 49:1, 1966.

52. N. B. Kurnick and P. A. Lindsay, Nucleic acids in compensatory renal hypertrophy, *Lab Invest* 18:700, 1968.

53. B. Zumoff and M. R. Pachter, Studies of rat kidney and liver growth using total nuclear counts, *Amer J Anat* 114:479, 1964.

54. G. E. G. Williams, Studies on the control of compensatory hyperplasia of the kidney in the rat, *Lab Invest* 11:1295, 1962.

55. C. E. McCreight and N. M. Sulkin, Compensatory renal hyperplasia following experimental surgical deletions of the kidney complement, *Amer J Anat* 110:199, 1962.

56. R. A. Malt and W. L. Miller, Sequential changes in classes of RNA during compensatory growth of the kidney, *J Exp Med* 126:1, 1967.

57. R. J. Reiter, Cellular proliferation and deoxyribonucleic acid synthesis in compensating kidneys of mice and the effect of food and water restriction, *Lab Invest* 14:1636, 1965.

58. I. Lieberman, R. Abrams, and P. Ove, Changes in the metabolism of ribonucleic acid preceding the synthesis of deoxyribonucleic acid in mammalian cells cultured from the animal, *J Biol Chem* 238:2141, 1963.

59. B. Mach and P. Vassalli, Biosynthesis of RNA in antibody-producing tissues, *Proc Nat Acad Sci USA* 54:975, 1965.

60. H. Kubinski and G. Koch, Regulation of the synthesis of various ribonucleic acids in animal cells, *Biochem Biophys Res Commun* 22:346, 1966.

61. L. L. MacKay, T. Addis, and E. M. MacKay, The degree of compensatory renal hypertrophy following unilateral nephrectomy. II. The influence of the protein intake, *J Exp Med* 67:515, 1938.

62. T. L. Phillips and L. W. Wachtel, Suppression of cellular proliferation in weanling rat kidneys by short-term fasting, *Proc Soc Exp Biol Med* 128:566, 1968.

63. R. A. Malt, Compensatory growth of the kidney, *New Eng J Med* 280:1446, 1969.

64. T. L. Phillips and G. F. Leong, Kidney cell proliferation after unilateral nephrectomy as related to age, *Cancer Res* 27:286, 1967.

65. E. M. MacKay, L. L. MacKay, and T. Addis, The degree of compensatory renal hypertrophy following unilateral nephrectomy. I. The influence of age, *J Exp Med* 56:255, 1932.

66. R. Karp, J. A. Brasel, and M. Winick, Compensatory kidney growth after uninephrectomy in adult and infant rats, *Amer J Dis Child* 121:186, 1971.

67. M. Winick and A. Noble, Cellular response in rats during malnutrition at various ages, *J Nutr* 89:300, 1966.

68. W. S. Kerr, Jr., Effects of complete ureteral obstruction in dogs on kidney function, *Amer J Physiol* 184:521, 1956.

69. L. Benitez and J. A. Shaka, Cell proliferation in experimental hydronephrosis and compensatory renal hyperplasia, *Amer J Path* 44:961, 1964.

70. D. P. Simpson, Hyperplasia after unilateral nephrectomy and role of excretory load in its production, *Amer J Physiol* 201:517, 1961.

71. P. C. Royce, Inhibition of renal growth following unilateral nephrectomy in the rat, *Proc Soc Exp Biol Med* 113:1046, 1963.

72. D. Eckert, S. L. Kountz, and R. Cohn, Inhibition of compensatory renal growth by ureterocaval fistula, *J Surg Res* 9:187, 1969.

73. M. Rabinovitch and S. R. Dohi, Increase in serum ribonuclease activity after bilateral nephrectomy, *Amer J Physiol* 187:525, 1956.

74. L. M. Lowenstein and A. Stern, Serum factor in renal compensatory hyperplasia, *Science* 142:1479, 1963.

75. N. B. Kurnick and P. A. Lindsay, Compensatory renal hypertrophy in parabiotic mice, *Lab Invest* 19:45, 1968.

76. H. A. Johnson and K. D. Knudsen, Renal efficiency and information theory, *Nature* (*London*) 206:930, 1965.

Index

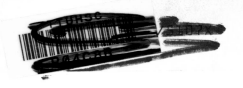

Date Due